KU-515-529

WARRINGTON AND HALTON HOSPITALS
NHS FOUNDATION TRUST
B09103

A SIMPLE GUIDE TO BLOOD GAS ANALYSIS

Normal ranges for blood gas analysis

Measure	Normal range
pH	7·36–7·44
$PaCO_2$	35–45 mmHg (4·7–6·0 kPa)
Actual HCO_3^-	21–28 mmol/l
Standard HCO_3^-	21–27 mmol/l
Base excess	±2 mmol/l
PaO_2	Over 90 mm Hg (12·0 kPa) on room air

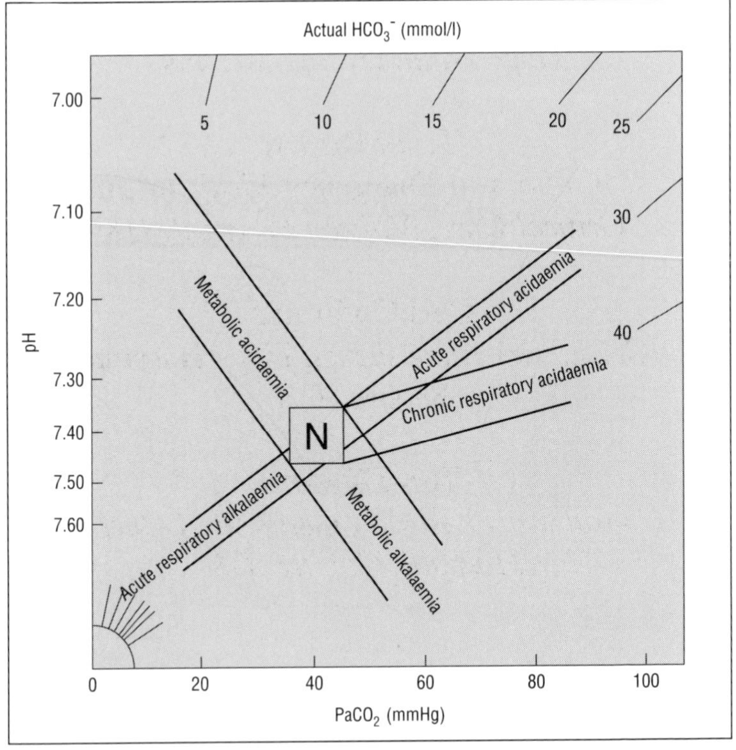

Acid-base nomogram in the interpretation of arterial blood gases.

A SIMPLE GUIDE TO BLOOD GAS ANALYSIS

Peter Driscoll
Senior Lecturer in Emergency Medicine, Hope Hospital, Salford, UK

Terry Brown
Consultant in Emergency Medicine and Critical Care, Whiston Hospital, UK

Carl Gwinnutt
Consultant Anaesthetist, Hope Hospital, Salford, UK

Terry Wardle
Consultant Physician, Countess of Chester Hospital, Chester, UK

Illustrations by
Bridget Landon

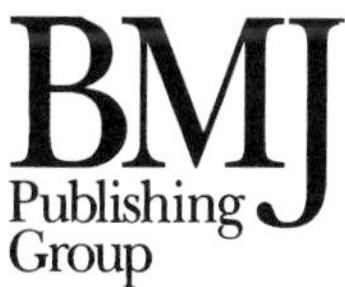

First published in 1997
Second impression 2000
by the BMJ Publishing Group, BMA House, Tavistock Square, London WC1H 9JR

British Library Cataloguing in Publication Data

A catalogue record for this book is available from the British Library

ISBN 0-7279-1107-4

Typeset by Apek Typesetters Ltd, Nailsea, Bristol
Printed and bound in Great Britain by Latimer Trend & Company Ltd, Plymouth

Contents

Acknowledgements

We are eternally grateful for all those people who gave helpful suggestions during the writing of this book. In particular we thank: Peter Baskett, Sarah Green, Roop Kishen, Gabby Lomas, Vanessa Lloyd-Davis, Graham McKinnon, Geraldine McMahon, David Nicholson, Peter Nightingale, Marie Noelle, Joan Sabir, Suki Sahir, Catherine Shaw, Helen Sinnott, Steve Southworth, Tony Thomas, Robin Touquet, Chris Ward, and Jill Windle.

Introduction

Why you should read this book

Blood gas analysis enables you to assess a patient's acid-base status as well as important aspects of their respiratory physiology. These two topics are infamous, however, for causing confusion and anxiety in readers of medical textbooks. Such feelings are aggravated further by well meaning teachers explaining these topics with numerous equations and complex graphs. It is therefore not surprising that when they come together in blood gas analysis, many students have problems.

Though an understanding of acid-base balance and respiratory physiology is required to interpret a blood gas result, the clinician does not require the brain power normally associated with landing a space probe on Mars! This book will show you how it is possible to achieve the following aims painlessly:

- An understanding of how the body regulates acid-base disturbances
- An understanding of relevant respiratory physiology
- A system of how to interpret a patient's blood gas results.

Style

This book is written for medical students, junior doctors (residents), and nursing staff dealing with patients whose management is being determined, in part, by analysis of their blood gas results. It is designed to enable you to enjoy reading about this subject at the same time as acquiring important information. To this end, equations are kept to the minimum and the Henderson-Hasselbach equation is not discussed. Instead principles are described in (we hope) conversational English, and cartoons and summaries are used frequently to reinforce crucial parts of the text.

Futhermore each chapter finishes with a self assessment quiz to enable you to test your understanding of the topics covered. In addition the answers are provided with a comprehensive description of the reasoning as well as relevant page references for further reading.

Layout

Chapters 1 to 4 provide you with a "survival guide" to blood gas analysis and assume no prior knowledge of acid-base balance, respiratory physiology, or blood gas interpretation. They therefore include descriptions of the technique of taking a blood gas sample, an explanation of common terminology, factors affecting oxygen uptake, and how the body regulates normal and abnormal changes in its acid-base balance. With these basic principles described you then have the opportunity to test your understanding when common acidoses and alkaloses are discussed in chapters 5 and 6.

All these points are brought together in the final chapter. In doing so it describes a system that will enable you to interpret results from an arterial blood gas sample.

This book is dedicated to Sue, Noel, and Harry.
Their professionalism made it all possible.

1 How to take an arterial blood gas sample

CARL GWINNUTT

Objectives

The objective of this chapter is to describe:

- The preparation required for taking an arterial sample
- How an arterial sample can be obtained
- Precautions to be taken when obtaining an arterial sample
- Helpful tips on how to overcome common problems.

An arterial sample can be obtained by either a percutaneous puncture of an artery or aspiration from an indwelling arterial cannula. If these samples are taken incorrectly, however, then any analysis will be invalid and, more importantly, the patient is at risk of being injured. This chapter will therefore describe the correct way of taking samples from both sources so that meaningful results can be obtained with minimal discomfort to the patient.

Obtaining a blood sample from an arterial puncture

Preparation

Sites of puncture

The site chosen for taking arterial blood depends on factors such as your own preference and skill, access, and the patient's clinical condition. The radial, brachial, and femoral arteries are three most commonly used, but it must be remembered that veins lie close by in each case. Consequently a venous blood sample can be obtained by mistake, particularly when a femoral approach is used.

Box 1.1 Contraindications to using the radial artery

- Absent ulnar circulation (figure 1.2)
- Impaired circulation in the hand (for example, Raynaud's disease or Buerger's disease)
- Underlying skeletal trauma
- An arteriovenous fistula for dialysis

The radial artery is used most often in conscious patients as access is easy. The artery is superficial (0·5–1·0 cm beneath the skin), and pressure is easily applied to arrest bleeding. Provided there are no contraindications (box 1.1) the needle is inserted at the point of maximum pulsation just proximal to the proximal transverse skin crease at the wrist (figure 1.1).

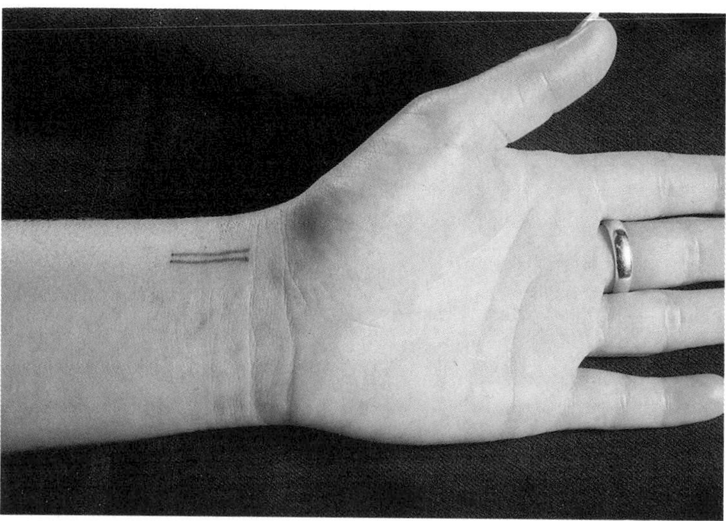

Figure 1.1 Surface anatomy—radial artery.

The brachial artery is used as an alternative to the radial artery but it is deeper (0·5–1·5 cm from the skin). Provided there are no contraindications (box 1.2) the needle is inserted medial to the biceps tendon over the point of maximum pulsation. It should be remembered that the median nerve lies medial to the artery (figure 1.3).

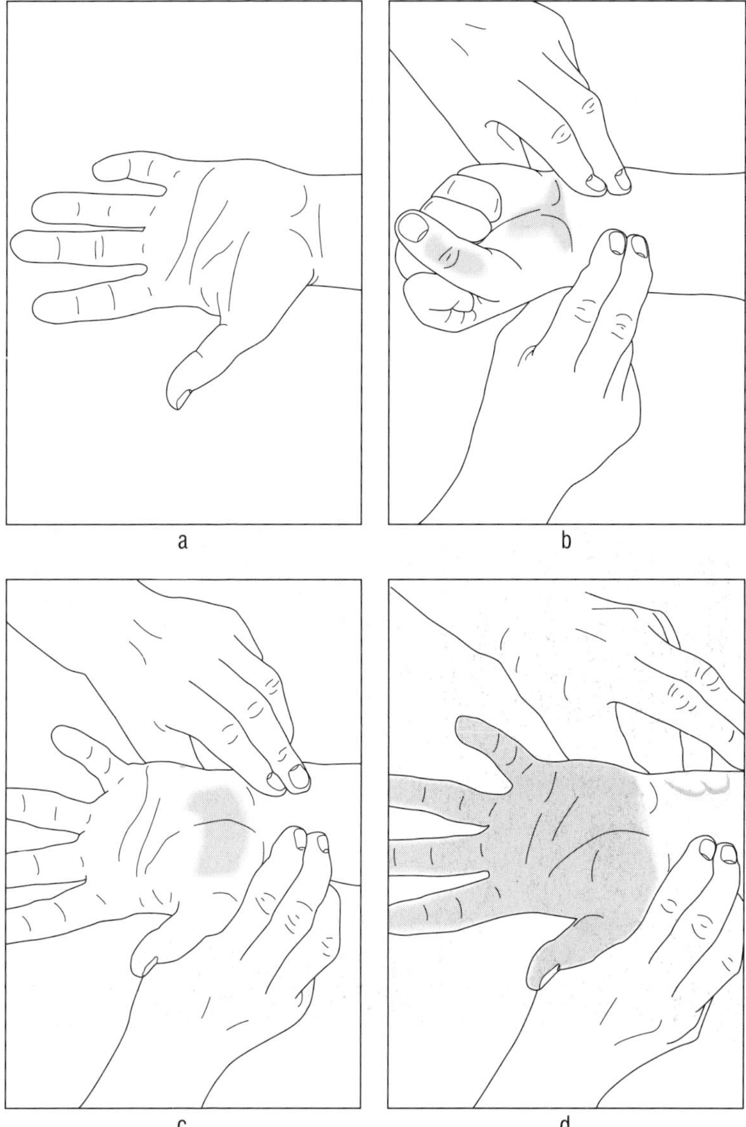

Figure 1.2 Allen's test. *a* Hand at rest; *b* patient clenches fist and hand, pressure is applied over radial and ulnar arteries; *c* as the arterial compression is maintained the hand is pale; *d* compression over ulnar artery is released. The distinct pink colouration of palm indicates that there is good ulnar circulation. Consequently puncture of the radial artery is not contraindicated in this patient.

Box 1.2 Contraindications to using the brachial artery

- Impaired circulation distally as damage may cause ischaemia because the brachial artery is an end artery
- Fracture around the elbow because of the risk of introducing infection
- An arteriovenous fistula in the forearm

The femoral artery is used when the above two sites have failed or the patient is shocked and the peripheral arteries are difficult to feel. It is the deepest of the three arteries described (2·0–4·0 cm from the skin) and lies between the femoral vein (medially) and the femoral nerve (laterally). Provided there are no contraindications (box 1.3) the needle is introduced at the mid-inguinal point, 2 cm below the inguinal ligament over the point of maximal pulsation (figure 1.4).

Equipment

Although little equipment is required to take an arterial blood sample, it should all be prepared beforehand (box 1.4). **Furthermore as with any technique where there is the risk of blood contact, gloves must be worn by the operator and assistant**.

The syringe must be adequately heparinised to prevent the sample clotting because this will cause the blood gas analyser to produce an erroneous result. As heparin is an acid, however, the minimum amount should be used to prevent artefacts. In practice, therefore, 0.25 ml of heparin (1000 IU/ml) is drawn up into the syringe. The plunger is then withdrawn to allow the heparin to coat

Box 1.3 Contraindications to using the femoral artery

- Extensive vascular disease because of the risk of dislodging a plaque, which may embolise distally
- When the artery has been replaced by a graft
- In children because of the risk of septic arthritis and nerve injury

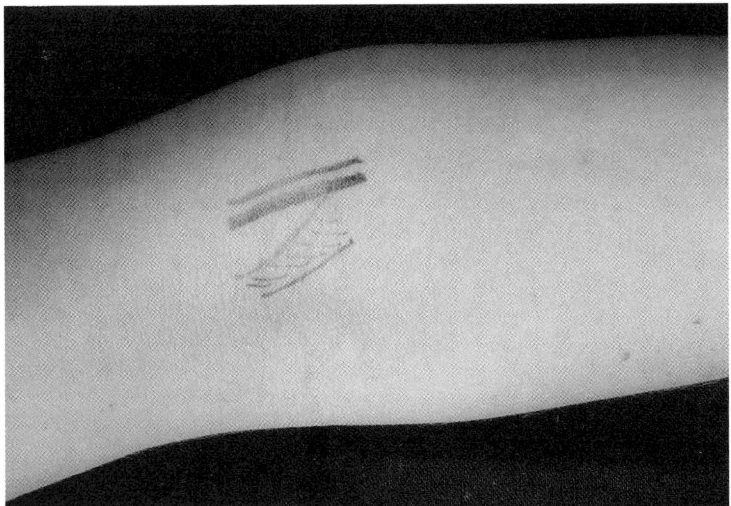

Figure 1.3 Surface anatomy—brachial artery.

the walls of the syringe and then the heparin is expelled completely. This leaves a small but adequate amount in the syringe and needle. Alternatively, a commercially prepared syringe already containing heparin can be used in a similar manner. These syringes also have

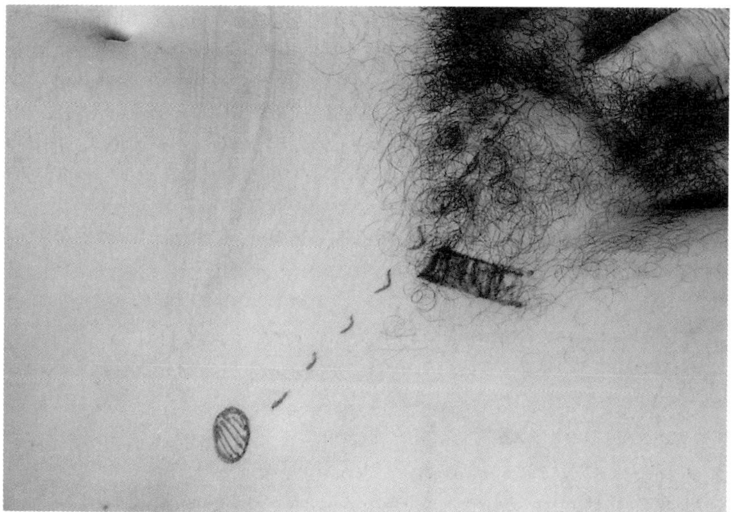

Figure 1.4 Surface anatomy—femoral artery.

Box 1.4 Equipment required for obtaining an arterial sample

- Skin preparation fluid–alcohol or iodine based
- Syringe size 2 ml containing 0.5% or 1% plain lignocaine (lidocaine) with a 25 g (orange) needle attached
- Needle size 23 g (blue) attached to a heparinised syringe for radial or brachial sampling or a 21 g (green) needle for femoral sampling
- Sharps' bin
- Gauze swabs or cotton wool for applying pressure on the puncture site after the sample has been taken
- Cap to seal syringe
- Ice if transportation to the laboratory will take over 5 minutes

a very low resistance plunger, which allows the syringe to fill under arterial pressure without the need for aspiration.

Procedure

Before starting it is essential to give the patient an explanation of what you are about to do and to obtain their verbal consent if possible. Then after you have assembled the equipment in a clean tray, the patient should be positioned according to the planned site of puncture. In the case of radial or brachial arterial samples the patient should lie semirecumbent on a bed with the chosen, non-dominant arm supported on a pillow. If the radial artery is to be used the wrist should be extended by 20–30° as this moves the artery into a more superficial position. The patient may find it difficult to maintain this position when the arterial stab is taking place. Therefore it is best to have the position maintained with the help of an assistant (figure 1.5). Alternatively, if you are working single handed, you can tape the patient's supine hand over a half litre bag of crystalloid. When the femoral artery is being used the patient should be supine on a bed or trolley.

Once the above tasks have been completed the following sequence of events should be carried out:

- Under aseptic conditions identify the pulse in the desired area, then clean appropriately and allow the agent to dry. Check the point of maximum pulsation and warn the patient that local anaesthetic is about to be injected and some stinging will be

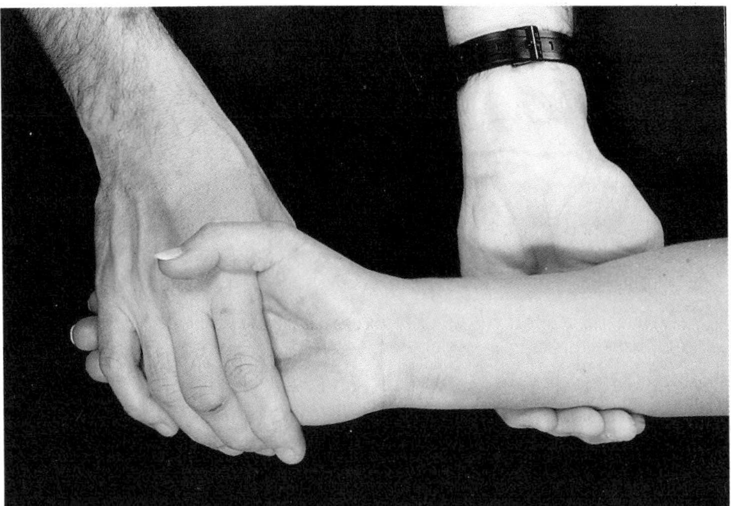

Figure 1.5 Assistant holding optimal position of wrist and not getting in operator's way.

felt.

- Subcutaneously infiltrate with the plain lignocaine (lidocaine), aspirating before injecting to ensure that you have not inadvertently entered a blood vessel (figure 1.6). Be careful not to use

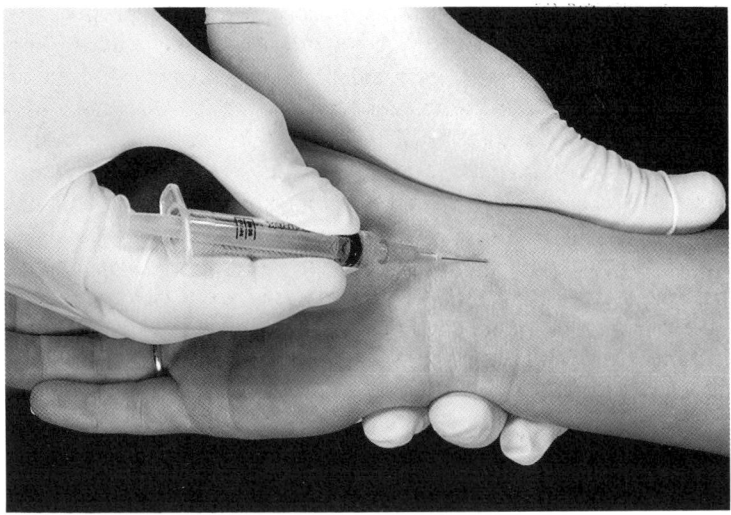

Figure 1.6 Infiltration with local anaesthetic.

too much local anaesthetic because this can obscure the location of the vessel. In practice 0·2–0·3 ml is sufficient for the radial, 0·4–0·6 ml for the brachial, and 0·6–1·0 ml for the femoral artery.

- Confirm the position of the artery with the fingers of your non-dominant hand (figure 1.7).
- Insert the needle, bevel facing upwards, towards the artery at an angle of 20°–30° to the horizontal for the radial and brachial arteries (figure 1.8) or 70° to the horizontal for the femoral artery.
- If a standard syringe is used, aspirate gently as the needle is advanced. This is not necessary for a low resistance type syringe.
- Aspirate 1–2 ml of blood and then withdraw the needle from the patient. You then need to remove the needle from the syringe safely and dispose of it in a sharps' bin. **Do not pass it to the assistant** because needle stick injuries can occur during this exchange. You can then cap the syringe and send it off for analysis. If you are on your own and are using one of the commercial packs, however, stick the needle into the provided plastic bung. This will prevent air getting into the syringe as you apply pressure to the arterial stab wound.

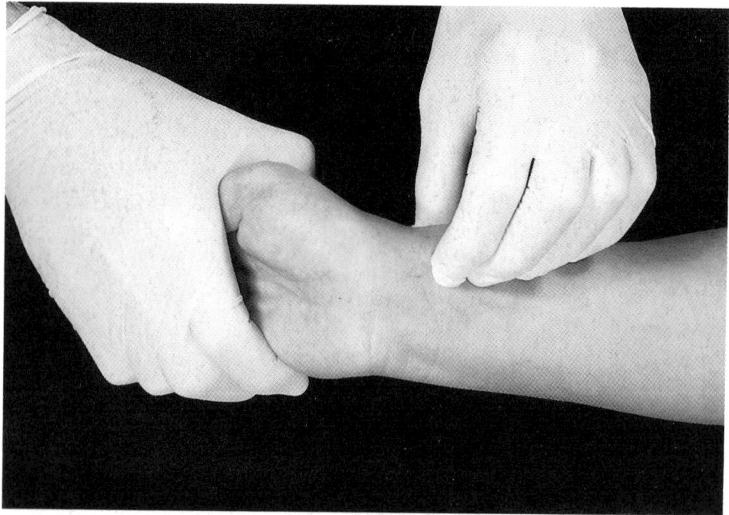

Figure 1.7 Confirming position of the artery with the fingers of the non-dominant hand.

- With cotton wool balls or gauze squares apply pressure to the puncture site for a minimum of 5 minutes before inspecting the area for swelling or bleeding. If either occur, reapply the pressure for a further 5 minutes.

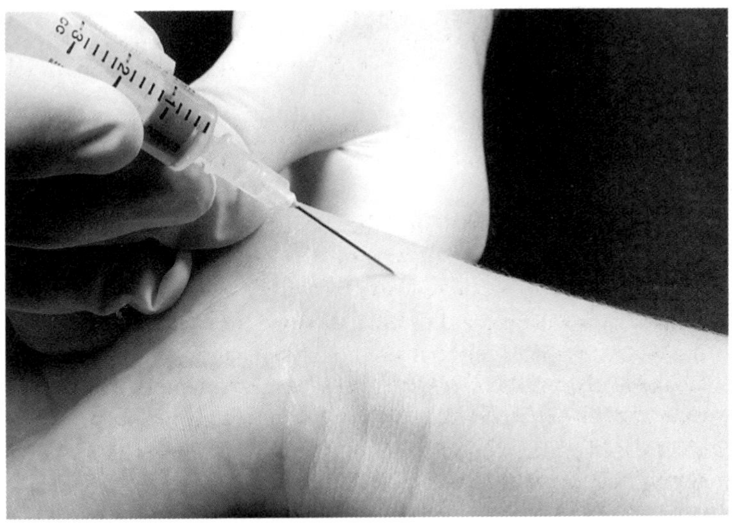

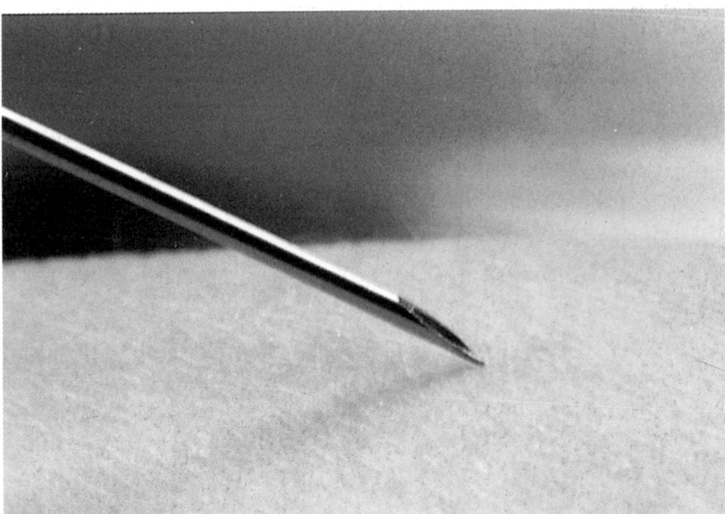

Figure 1.8 Inserting needle into the radial artery bevel upwards at an angle of 30° (lower photograph shows detail).

Precautions

If no blood is obtained after the needle has been inserted an appropriate distance it should be withdrawn slowly as it may have passed through the artery. Withdrawing the needle in this way will allow the tip to enter the lumen of the artery and a blood sample to be obtained.

If the patient complains of pain shooting distally a nerve may have been hit. Remove the needle completely and retry in a different direction.

Sluggish filling of the syringe usually indicates that you have accidently entered a vein rather than an artery. In this case remove the needle and after a few minutes of pressure try again.

> **Halt: Key point**
>
> **It is important to realise that you cannot use the colour of the sample to determine if it is arterial or venous. This is especially so if the patient is known or suspected to have a low level of oxygen in the circulation or is polycythaemic**

Obtaining a blood sample from an indwelling arterial cannula

Indwelling arterial cannulae are usually found in the same sites as already described for arterial punctures. Although it is easier to get an arterial sample from a cannula, there is no room for complacency. Gloves must be worn and a 5 ml syringe is needed in addition to one heparinised in the manner describe previously.

Once these precautions and preparations have been completed the following procedures should be carried out:

- Access to the cannula is usually via a three way tap. Attach a sterile, empty 5 ml syringe to the side port of the three way tap.
- Turn the tap to connect the artery to the syringe and remove 5 ml of blood (figure 1.9). This ensures that the subsequent sample is fresh blood and not diluted by the flushing solution between the tap and the artery.
- Turn off the tap, remove the syringe, and dispose of it appropriately.
- Attach the heparinised syringe, turn the tap back on, and very gently aspirate 1·0–2·0 ml of blood (figure 1.10).

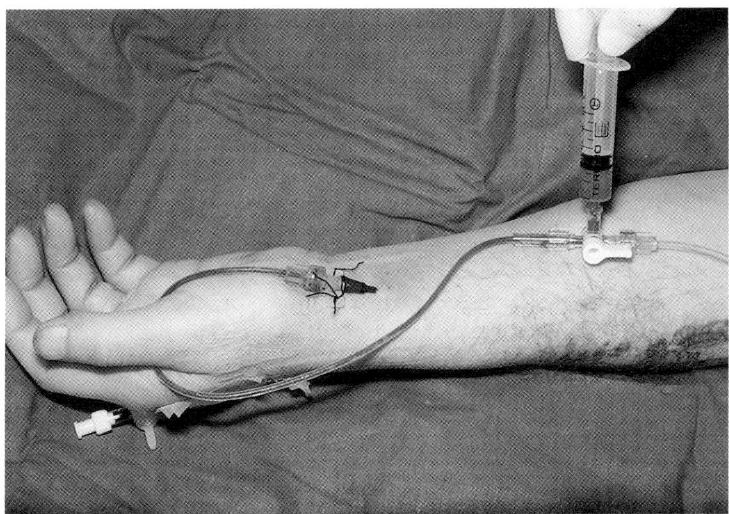

Figure 1.9 Syringe connected to the arterial cannula with 5 ml of blood being withdrawn.

- Turn off the tap, and remove and cap the syringe.
- Flush the port on the tap into a receiver, and then finish by squirting some flushing solution through the cannula to ensure that the system does not become blocked by clot.

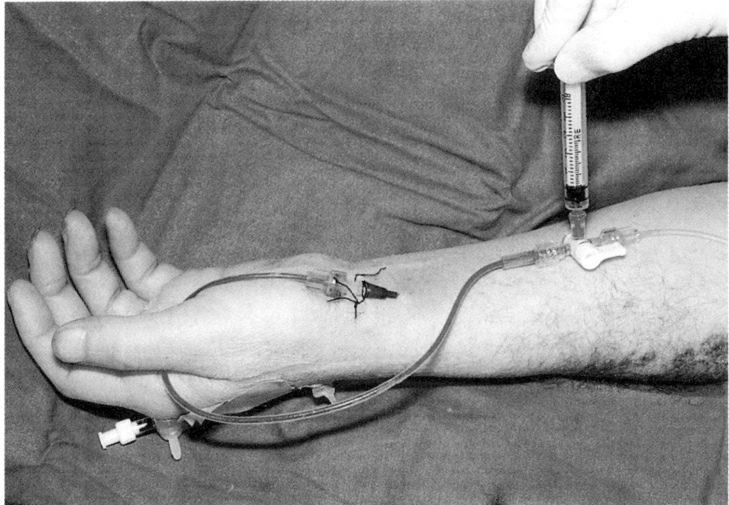

Figure 1.10 Aspiration of 1·0–2·0 ml of blood.

Handy hints to avoid common errors

There are several common iatrogenic errors made when arterial blood gas samples are obtained. These can be avoided by considering the following points:

- The concentrations of the gases in the sample will be affected if the posture of critically ill patients changes, the composition of the inspired gas is altered, or the breathing pattern is altered. It is therefore important to take the sample 3–5 minutes after any such changes so that an accurate reading can be obtained while a steady state has been achieved. As equilibration with the inspired gas is slower in patients with pulmonary disease a longer time interval should be given before the sample is taken.*
- Warn the laboratory that you are sending an arterial sample—they may be servicing their blood gas analyser. If you are performing the analysis yourself make sure the machine is available, calibrated daily, subjected to regular quality control, and you know how to use it.
- Carefully expel any obvious air bubbles from the sample and seal the syringe. This is particularly important if a long transportation time to the laboratory is expected. Failure to do this will allow oxygen and carbon dioxide to diffuse in or out of the sample from the bubbles and so alter their concentrations within minutes.
- You need to keep the sample in melting ice if a transport time of over 5 minutes is expected. This slows down any metabolic activity of the cells, which may affect the result.
- Clearly mark any hazardous samples, and fill in the request form accurately. **This must include the patient's inspired oxygen concentration**. The latter is essential for the interpretation of the results, and it will also enable the laboratory staff to check the validity of their analyser. Clinical history, results of physical examination, medication, recent bicarbonate administration, full blood count, and electrolyte screen should also have been noted because these allow you to put the results into clinical context.
- If a sample of arterial blood is taken from a hypothermic patient and warmed to 37·0 °C by the blood gas machine, then gas solubility will decrease. This will result in a false increase of the carbon dioxide and oxygen readings as well as a false reduction in the pH. Some authorities suggest, therefore, that the results of

* In patients with chronic pulmonary conditions it can take up to 30 minutes to reach a steady state after changes are made.

blood gas sampling should be corrected for the temperature of the patient. Although theoretically this gives a more accurate picture of the patient's status, the current consensus is that uncorrected results should be used to guide treatment for acid-base disturbances in patients with hypothermia.

- If at first you don't succeed in obtaining an arterial sample, don't keep trying. As taking samples is painful, it makes the patient hyperventilate and means that you don't get a truly representative result. The answer is quite simple—get help!

Summary

Before an arterial bood gas sample is interpreted it is essential that it is obtained appropriately so that it is free of any iatrogenic errors. This requires preparation and the carrying out of the procedure in a safe and effective way. The sample should then be sent as quickly as possible to a blood gas analyser, which is calibrated daily and subjected to regular quality control.

Quiz

This chapter has discussed how to take an arterial blood sample. Go for a walk and think for a few minutes about what you have read. When you come back take the opportunity to test your comprehension by attempting quiz 1 below:

Quiz 1 (answers on page 150)

1. **Which are the three commonest sites for arterial puncture, and which lies closest to the skin surface?**
2. **What are the contraindications to using a radial artery for arterial puncture?**
3. **What lies medial to the femoral artery in the groin?**
4. **Why should the syringes that are used to collect the arterial sample be heparinised?**
5. **What effect can heparin have on the arterial sample?**
6. **What are the angles for inserting a needle into the brachial and femoral arteries?**
7. **When would you suspect that you have taken a venous sample by mistake?**
8. **How much blood should be removed from an indwelling arterial cannula before an arterial sample is taken for blood gas analysis?**

9 How often should a blood gas analyser be calibrated?

10 When should the arterial sample be kept on ice?

2 Useful terminology

PETER DRISCOLL

Objective

- To explain the meaning of commonly used terms in blood gas analysis and acid-base balance.

It is important to have a clear understanding of what is meant by the commonly used terms in blood gas analysis and acid-base balance. For ease of reference therefore this chapter provides explanations of most of the terms used in this book (box 2.1). As the reading of terminology chapters requires concentration and stamina, however, we suggest that you attempt the following questions and see how many terms you are already familiar with. Using the page references with each answer you can then concentrate on relevant parts of the chapter before rechecking your knowledge with the same test on page 36.

Box 2.1 Common terms described in this chapter

- Concentrations
- Normal ranges
- Acids, bases, and alkalis
- pH scale, acidaemia, and alkalaemia
- Acidosis and alkalosis
- Buffers
- Buffer saturation
- Standard and actual bicarbonate
- Base excess and base deficit
- Ventilation and respiration

Quiz 2 (this is repeated at the end of this chapter on page 36; the answers are on page 150–2)

1. How many milligrams of sodium chloride are there in 10 ml of a 1 molar solution?
2. How much lignocaine (lidocaine) is there in 10 ml of a 2% solution?
3. What is the partial pressure of carbon dioxide in dry air at sea level?
4. What is the partial pressure of nitrogen in dry air at sea level?
5. What does PaO_2 mean?
6. What is 40 mm Hg expressed in kPa?
7. What is the difference between an acidaemia and an acidosis?
8. What is the difference between a base and an alkali?
9. Name an intracellular and extracellular buffer?
10. What does a base excess of −6 mmol/l mean?

Concentrations

Every day in our clinical practice we deal with concentrations. We use these numbers as an indication of how much of a substance is dissolved in solution. As an example consider the following common solutions:

- A 1 molar solution is the molecular weight of a substance (in grams) in each litre.
- 1% Lignocaine is 1 g of lignocaine (lidocaine) per 100 ml of saline.
- 5% Dextrose is 5 g of dextrose per 100 ml of water.
- 1:1000 Adrenaline is 1 g of adrenaline per 1000 ml of saline.
- 1:10 000 Adrenaline is 1 g of adrenaline per 10 000 ml of saline.

Molar solution

Molar units are commonly used to describe the concentration of electrolytes in a solution. For example, a molar solution of sodium chloride would contain the molecular weight of sodium chloride in grams in each litre of fluid. This is equal to 58.4 grams, because the gram molecular weights of sodium and chlorine are 23 and 35.4, respectively. When dealing with the small concentrations normally found in the human body, however, we have to use parts of a mole (table 2.1).

Molar solutions are used because the gram molecular weight of

Table 2.1 Common molar concentration units

Mole	Definition	Abbreviation	
Mole	Molecular weight of substance (in grams) in each litre	mol	1 M
Millimole	A thousandth of a mole	mmol	10^{-3} M
Micromole	A millionth of a mole	µmol	10^{-6} M
Nanomole	A billionth of a mole	nmol	10^{-9} M

any compound has the same number of molecules (6×10^{23} molecules to be precise!). Therefore, if we compare the molar solutions of two compounds we are in fact comparing the same number of molecules in each case.

Percentages

When dealing with a mixture of gases we tend to use percentages. For example, consider the room air you are breathing at the moment. Assuming it does not contain any water vapour, nearly 21% of each litre (that is, 210 ml) will be made up of oxygen while the remainder is nearly all nitrogen (box 2.2).

In clinical practice we can increase the proportion of inspired oxygen up to 100%. In these circumstances the oxygen concentration is expressed as a fraction (FIO_2). For example, an FIO_2 of 0·5 would mean the patient was breathing a gas that was 50% oxygen. Similarly an FIO_2 of 0·85 would mean the patient was breathing a gas that was 85% oxygen.

Entonox is a mixture of gases that is commonly used in clinical practice to provide pain relief. This gas is made up of 50% oxygen and 50% nitrous oxide—that is, half of every litre of this gas is oxygen and the other half is nitrous oxide.

Percentages on their own, however, do not tell how much of a gas is present—that is, its concentration. To illustrate this point consider the following example (figure 2.1). Both containers have

Box 2.2 Composition of dry air

- Nitrogen 78·06%
- Oxygen 20·98%
- Carbon dioxide 00·04%
- Inert gases 00·92%

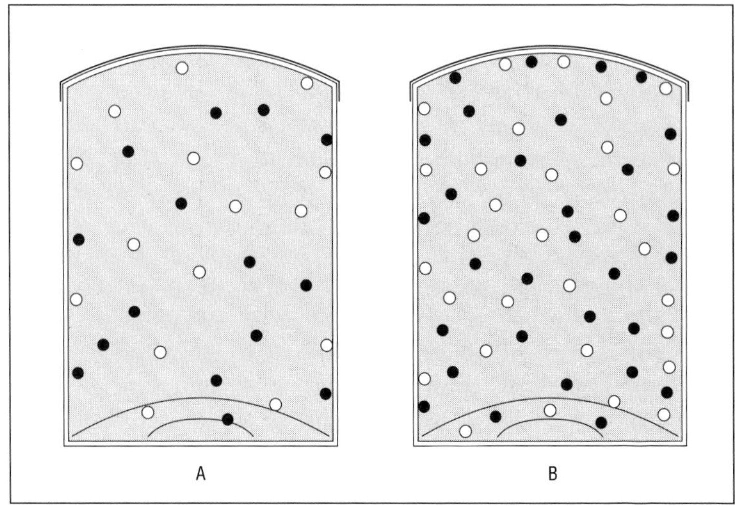

Figure 2.1 Two containers with different number of molecules in each. They can have the same percentage volume but different amounts of gas in each case.

gases that are 50% oxygen and 50% nitrogen. B, however, has twice the number of molecules as A. Therefore to determine how much of a gas is present we need to know, in addition to its percentage, the number of molecules present. As physically counting molecules is not possible we need to look for a way of estimating how many molecules are present. We do this by measuring the partial pressure of the gas.

Partial pressure

The pressure of any gas is the sum total of the molecules in the gas colliding with the walls of its container (figure 2.2). If the gas is a mixture (such as air) then the total pressure is the sum of all the individual gas pressures:

Total pressure of air = pressure of (nitrogen + oxygen + carbon dioxide + inert gases)

Which is:

$$760 = 593{\cdot}2 + 159 + 0{\cdot}3 + 6{\cdot}9$$

The pressure of an individual gas is known as its partial pressure. This is usually indicated by the letter "P"—for example, PO_2 indicates the partial pressure of oxygen.

The partial pressure of any particular gas in a mixture can be

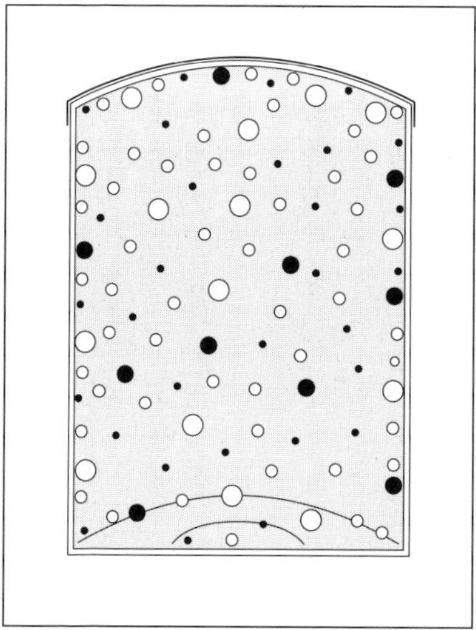

Figure 2.2 Pressure of a gas mixture is the sum total of all the individual partial pressures as a result of the different molecules hitting the side.

calculated by multiplying the percentage of that gas divided by 100 (this is called the **fraction** of the gas), by the total pressure of the mixture. For example the partial pressure of oxygen in dry air at sea level is:

$$20{\cdot}98/100 \times 760 = 159 \text{ mm Hg}$$

where 20·98 is the percentage of oxygen in air and 760 mm Hg is the atmospheric pressure at sea level (that is, the total pressure of air).

When a gas mixture is in contact with a liquid, some of the gas will dissolve in the liquid (figure 2.3). The volume that dissolves depends on two things: the partial pressure of the individual gas forcing the molecules into the liquid, and the ease of the individual gas molecules to get into the liquid (that is, its solubility). For example, carbon dioxide is 20 times more soluble in plasma than oxygen. Therefore, more CO_2 than oxygen will dissolve in plasma for any given partial pressure.

In time, provided the gas and solution are left undisturbed, an equilibrium will develop whereby the number of molecules of gas leaving the liquid will equal the number entering the liquid (figure 2.4). At this point the partial pressure of each individual gas within the liquid will be equal to the partial pressure of the same gas in

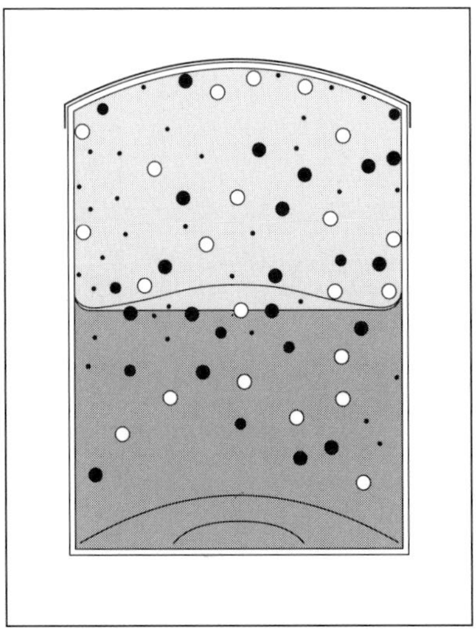

Figure 2.3 Interface between liquid and gas medium. Container shows molecules moving into and out of the liquid.

contact with the liquid. To avoid confusion therefore it is important to indicate the medium in which the partial pressure of the gas was measured. This is written as Pmedium. If we take oxygen as an example:

PO_2 = partial pressure of oxygen in the atmosphere

PAO_2 = partial pressure of oxygen in the alveoli

PaO_2 = partial pressure of oxygen in arterial blood

PvO_2 = partial pressure of oxygen in venous blood

In a healthy person breathing room air the normal partial pressures of carbon dioxide and oxygen in an arterial blood sample are:

$PaCO_2$ = 35–45 mm Hg (4·7–6·0 kPa)

PaO_2 = over 90 mm Hg (over 12·0 kPa)

As demonstrated above there are two types of units used to measure pressures—millimetres of mercury (mm Hg) or kilopascals (kPa). In the United States and many hospitals in the United Kingdom mm Hg are still used. In continental Europe, however, there is a move to replace these with kPa. In this book we will use both throughout, but if you want to convert one to the other the formula is:

$$1 \text{ kPa} = 7{\cdot}5 \text{ mm Hg}$$

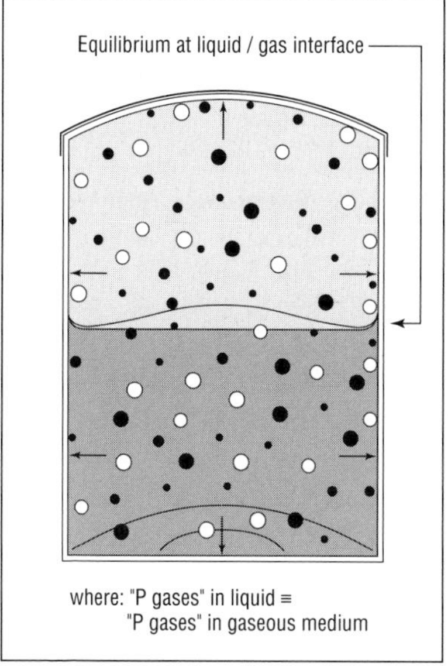

Figure 2.4 Equilibrium between liquid and gas. Container shows the same number of molecules of various size moving into and out of the liquid. The partial pressures of the individual gases are the same in the liquid and in the gas.

Halt: Key points

- **The partial pressure of a gas is a measure of the concentration of the gas in the medium it is in (for example, arterial blood)**
- **The partial pressure and solubility of a gas govern how many molecules of the gas will dissolve in a liquid it is in contact with**
- **You need to indicate the medium from which the sample was taken (for example, Pa = partial pressure in an arterial blood sample)**
- **Partial pressures are measured in either mm Hg or kPa**

Normal ranges

When the same biochemical variable is compared among normal people it is common to find a range of values. For example, the normal range for sodium is 135–150 mmol/l. Some of this variation is due to the differences between the machines used to measure the variable. The biggest cause for the range of values, however, is that people are different (even normal ones!). Factors such as age, sex, medical history, and medication can all affect biochemical parameters.

Most normal ranges are chosen arbitrarily to include 95% of the values found in healthy volunteers. By definition therefore, 5% of the normal population will have values outside this range. Nevertheless, the further the result is away from the normal range the more likely it is to be pathological.

In this book the normal ranges described are based on healthy adult volunteers who are not taking any medication and have no significant previous medical problems.*

Acids, bases, and alkalis

Originally the word acid was used to describe the sour taste of unripe fruit. Subsequently many other different meanings have been attributed to it, and this has led to considerable confusion and misunderstanding. To overcome these difficulties, the modern definition is based on the chemical properties of a substance. As a result an acid is defined as any substance that is capable of providing hydrogen ions (H^+) when it is a solution.

It follows that a strong acid is a substance that will readily provide many hydrogen ions, and, conversely, a weak acid is a substance that provides only a few. An example of a strong acid normally found in the body is hydrochloric acid. This is produced by the cells lining the stomach. Elsewhere in the body there are many other types of acids, but these are all much weaker (box 2.3).

The opposite of an acid is a base, and this is defined as any substance that accepts hydrogen ions when it is in a solution. The stronger the base is the more readily it takes up hydrogen ions. As with acids the body is capable of producing a range of bases with most of them being weak (box 2.4). You will notice that proteins

* A variety of machines have been used to analyse the samples in this book. In all cases the machines, as well as the staff involved, met with nationally agreed laboratory analytical performance.

Box 2.3 Acids produced by the body

- Hydrochloric acid
- Lactic acid
- Carbonic acid
- Ketoacids
- Pyruvic acid
- Uric acid
- Proteins

can be either acids or bases. This is because they are made up of a long chain of molecules that can either provide or accept hydrogen ions.

Halt: Key points

- **An acid is any substance that is capable of providing H^+**
- **A base is any substance that is capable of accepting H^+**

An alkali is a substance that can donate hydroxide ions (OH^-). As it can also accept hydrogen ions, it therefore represents a particular type of base. Consequently sodium hydroxide (NaOH) is both an alkali and a base because it donates hydroxide ions and accepts hydrogen ions. It is therefore correct to say:

"all alkalis are bases but not all bases are alkalis!"

The pH scale, acidaemia, and alkalaemia

The concentration of hydrogen ions in any particular body fluid will determine how acidic it is. Normally in the blood this concentration is in the order of 0·000 000 04 mol/l or alternatively 40 nanomole/litre (nmol/l). To gain a perspective on how tiny this

Box 2.4 Bases produced by the body

- Bicarbonate
- Phosphate
- Proteins
- Ammonia

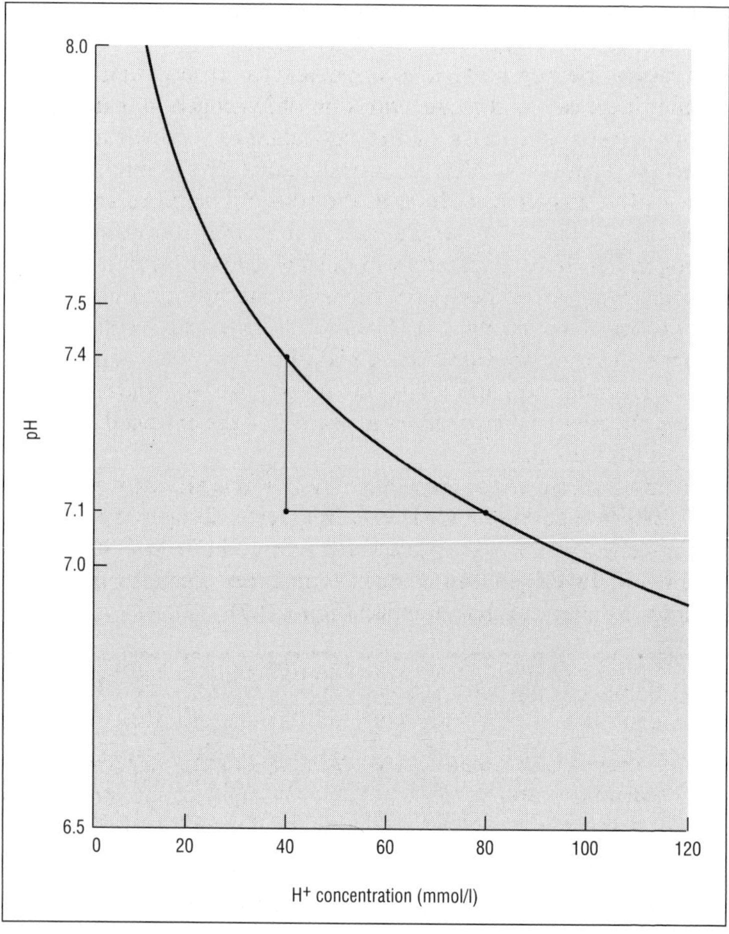

Figure 2.5 Relation between pH and hydrogen ion concentration, showing that when the pH goes from 7·4 to 7·1 the hydrogen ion concentration increases by 100%—that is, it goes from 40 to 80 nmol/l.

is, compare it with the concentration of other commonly measured electrolytes. For example, the plasma concetration of sodium is 0·135–0·145 mol/l—that is, 3 million times greater!

Dealing with such very small numbers is obviously difficult. Consequently in 1909 the pH scale was developed to express the concentration of hydrogen ions in a more convenient way. The normal pH of an arterial blood sample is between 7·36 and 7·44, and this is equivalent to a hydrogen ion concentration of 44–36 nmol/l respectively (figure 2.5); 6·8–7·8 is the pH range usually considered compatible with life. This is equivalent to a hydrogen ion concentration of 160–16 nmol/l.

In using the pH scale it is important to realise that the pH number increases as the concentration of hydrogen ions decreases and conversely decreases as the concentation of hydrogen ions increases (figure 2.5). This is a consequence of the mathematical process that was used to develop the scale.* Therefore an arterial blood pH below 7.36 would mean that the concentration of hydrogen ions had increased from normal. This condition is called an acidaemia, and it has many causes, some of which can be life threatening. Conversely, a pH above 7·44 would result from a reduction in the concentration of hydrogen ions. This condition is called an alkalaemia, and it also has several causes. Acidaemia and alkalaemia refer to disturbances in the pH of the extracellular fluid (for example, blood).

Another consequence of the derivation of the pH scale is the fact that small changes in pH mean relatively large changes in hydrogen ion concentration. For example, a fall in the pH from 7·40 to 7·10 means the hydrogen ion concentration has risen from 40 to 80 nmol/l—that is, it has doubled (figure 2.5).

Halt: Key points

- **Hydrogen ions are present in the body in only very low concentrations**
- **As the hydrogen ion concentration increases the pH falls**
- **As the hydrogen ion concentration falls the pH rises**
- **An acidaemia occurs when the pH falls below 7·36 and an alkalaemia when it rises above 7·44**
- **Small changes in the pH scale represent large changes in the concentration of hydrogen ions**

Acidosis and alkalosis

Acidosis and alkalosis are the terms used to describe the main source of the acid-base disturbance. They refer to processes occurring at a cellular level that, if left uncorrected, would result in pH changes—that is, an acidaemia or an alkalaemia (table 2.2).

* If you are interested, the pH is the negative logarithm of the hydrogen ion concentration. Still interested?

Table 2.2 Acidosis and alkalosis

Type	The main disorder
Metabolic acidosis	A decrease in bicarbonate
Metabolic alkalosis	An increase in bicarbonate
Respiratory acidosis	An increase in carbon dioxide
Respiratory alkalosis	A decrease in carbon dioxide

Many people use the term "acidosis" to refer to an acidaemia and, similarly, the term "alkalosis" to refer to an alkalaemia. This is incorrect because the terms acidosis and alkalosis may still apply even if the pH is normal. For example, a patient may be simultaneously producing excessive but equal amounts of both acid and base such that they balance each other out. In this case the pH of an arterial sample would be within the normal range (that is, there is no acidaemia or alkalaemia) but the underlying pathological processes (that is, acidosis and alkalosis) would still be present. Therefore simply considering the pH alone may cause you to miss an underlying problem.

Do not be upset if you found the last paragraph a bit of a puzzle. Read through it again and take a minute to consider the points made. Once you feel it has been mastered, test your comprehension with the following phrase:

> **"You can have an acidosis without having an acidaemia but you cannot have an acidaemia without an acidosis!"**

Buffers

All of the complex chemical reactions occurring at a cellular level are controlled by special proteins called enzymes, which can function effectively at only very narrow ranges of pH. During normal activity, however, the body produces relatively larger amounts of hydrogen ions. Clearly something has to be done to prevent these hydrogen ions causing significant changes in pH before they are eliminated from the body. This is the function of buffers because within seconds they act to "take up" the free hydrogen ions both in the blood stream and in the cells of the body. Alternatively, when they are confronted with a strong base, they will give up hydrogen ions so that again a normal pH range can be maintained (figure 2.6).

Three quarters of the body's buffering power comes from proteins and organic phosphates located within the cells. Haemo-

H+ IONS
R
WIMPS
BUFFERS
R
FAB
DOWN
WITH
BASES
BUFF
BUFF
BUFFE
R
US

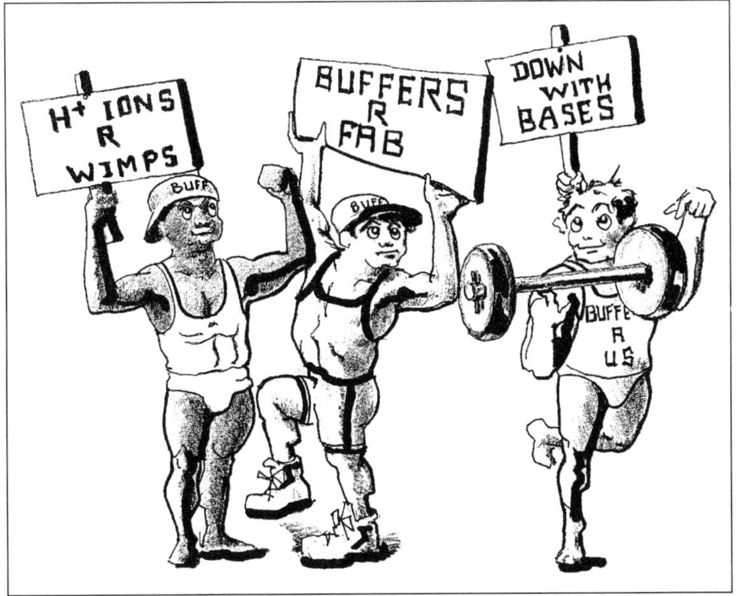

Figure 2.6

globin represents a particularly important type of intracellular protein buffer because it is very effective at both donating and accepting hydrogen ions when appropriate. It is also present in large amounts in the circulation. Extracellular buffers, in particular plasma proteins and the carbonic acid-bicarbonate system, make up the remaining quarter of the body's buffering power (box 2.5).*

The proteins act like big sponges that "soak up" the free

Box 2.5 Extracellular buffers

- Proteins (for example, albumin)
- Carbonic acid-bicarbonate system
- Phosphates (see footnote)
- Ammonia (in renal tubules)

* Phosphates are of little importance in the blood stream because their concentration in the extracellular fluid is only one twelfth that of the carbonic acid-bicarbonate system. In contrast they have a big buffering effect inside the cell because the concentration is much higher.

hydrogen ions and transport them to their place of elimination from the body. In most cases this is in the kidneys. In contrast, the carbonic acid-bicarbonate system acts by allowing the extra hydrogen ions to react with bicarbonate to produce carbon dioxide and water:

$$\underset{\text{Hydrogen ion}}{H^+} + \underset{\text{Bicarbonate ion}}{HCO_3^-} \leftrightarrow \underset{\text{Carbonic acid}}{H_2CO_3} \leftrightarrow \underset{\text{Carbon dioxide}}{CO_2} + \underset{\text{Water}}{H_2O}$$

The carbon dioxide is subsequently removed by the lungs. In so doing the additional free hydrogen ions are eliminated, allowing the pH to remain in its normal range.

The inorganic matrix of bone has vast quantities of sodium, potassium, and calcium that can be exchanged for hydrogen ions. As this removes the acid (or base) load from the circulation, bone can therefore provide a large buffering capacity. Though this takes longer to become effective it becomes particularly important in chronic acidotic states and when other extracellular buffer concentrations are low.

Buffer saturation

If you think of plasma proteins as large sponges that mop up hydrogen, it is easy to imagine them becoming "saturated" when they are dealing with an excessive acid load (figure 2.7). In this situation the plasma proteins will no longer be able to act as buffers until their abnormal acid load is removed in the normal manner—that is, mainly by the kidneys.

This problem of saturation does not apply to the carbonic acid-bicarbonate buffer system because the reaction between hydrogen and bicarbonate ions does not finish with carbonic acid. To understand why this should prevent saturation we need to consider this buffer system in a bit more detail.

From the description in the previous section we know that in the carbonic acid-bicarbonate buffer system hydrogen and bicarbonate ions come together to form carbonic acid. This acid then breaks down to form carbon dioxide and water:

$$H^+ + HCO_3^- \leftrightarrow H_2CO_3 \leftrightarrow CO_2 + H_2O$$

In the body there are literally billions of hydrogen and bicarbonate ions and carbon dioxide and water molecules.* Consequently billions of reactions are occurring at any one time. It

* For those of you who like numbers the actual figure is around 7×10^{26}!

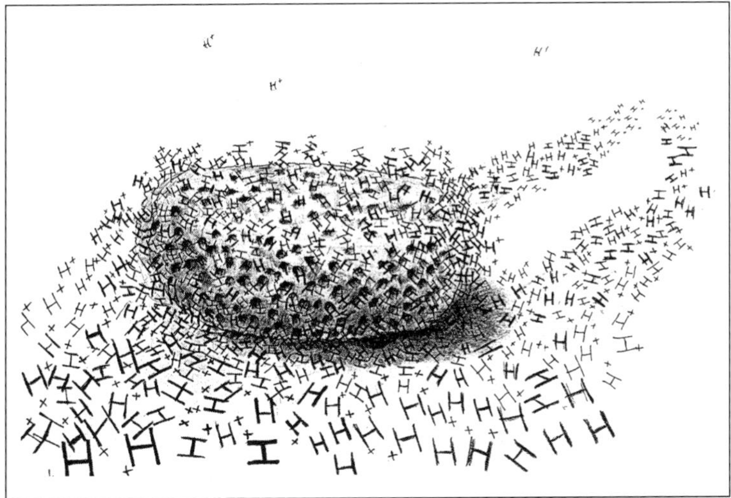

Figure 2.7 The protein "sponge" mops up a big puddle of hydrogen ions and becomes saturated.

is also important to realise that the symbol ↔ means that the reaction is capable of moving in either direction. In other words at any one time some molecules (that is, hydrogen and bicarbonate ions) are coming together such that the reaction moves to the right whereas others (that is, carbon dioxide and water) are coming together such that the reaction moves to the left (figure 2.8). The net effect in the body is therefore decided by the difference between the number of individual reactions moving to the left and the number of individual reactions moving to the right (figure 2.9).

Now let's consider the left hand side of the equation:

$$H^+ + HCO_3^- \leftrightarrow H_2CO_3$$

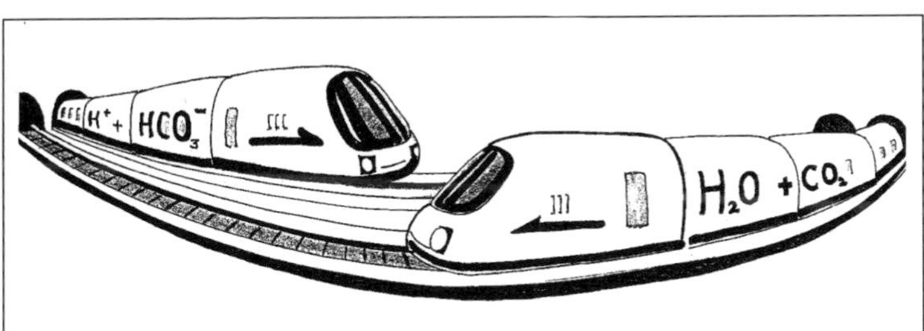

Figure 2.8

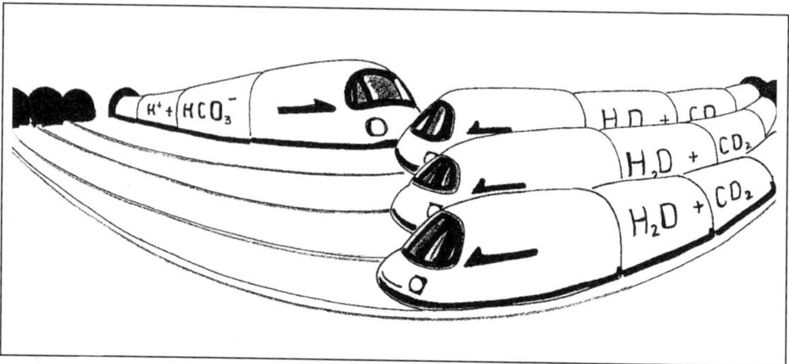

Figure 2.9

Carbonic acid is being continuously formed from hydrogen and bicarbonate ions at the same time as some carbonic acid molecules break down into bicarbonate and hydrogen ions (figure 2.10). There are, however, many more hydrogen and bicarbonate ions than carbonic acid molecules. Consequently the direction of the reaction is mainly to the right (that is, there is much more carbonic

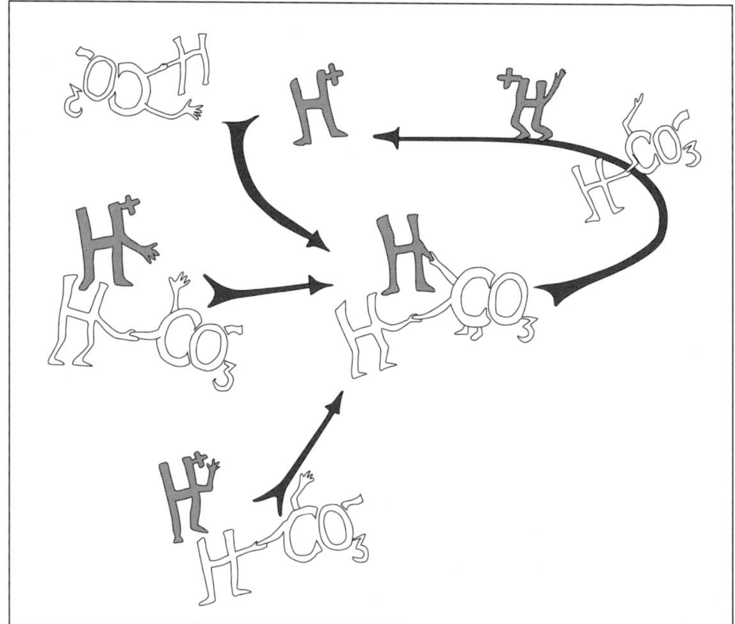

Figure 2.10 Simultaneous formation and breakdown of carbonic acid.

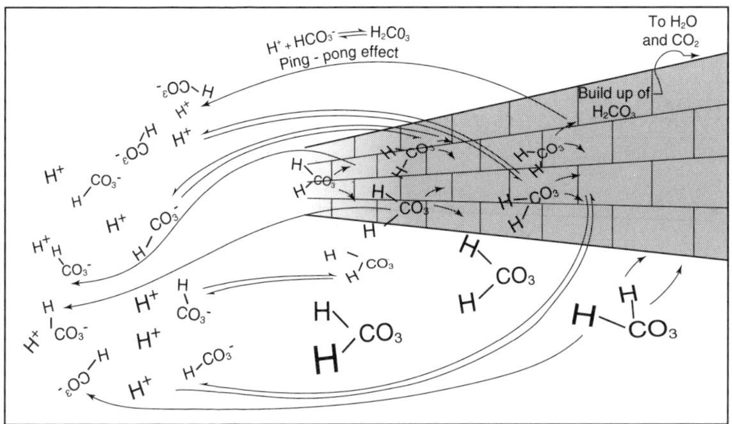

Figure 2.11 The build up of carbonic acid pushes the equation back to the left.

acid being formed than being broken down).

If carbonic acid could not break down into water and carbon dioxide the concentration of the acid would continue to build up (figure 2.11). As it did so the number of acid molecules breaking down into hydrogen and bicarbonate ions would increase. Eventually it would get so big that the amount of carbonic acid being formed would equal the amount of the acid being broken down into hydrogen ions and bicarbonate. This is known as a state of equilibrium because the movement to the right of the equation is equal to the movement to the left.

Halt: Key point

A state of equilibrium in the carbonic acid-bicarbonate buffer is when the net movement to the right is equal to the net movement to the left

If a state of equilibrium was allowed to occur, the carbonic acid-bicarbonate buffer system would be fully saturated. In real life, however, carbonic acid breaks down to carbon dioxide and water. Consequently, even when there is an excess of hydrogen ions—that is, pushing the equation to the right—carbonic acid does not accumulate. As a result of this low concentration of carbonic acid

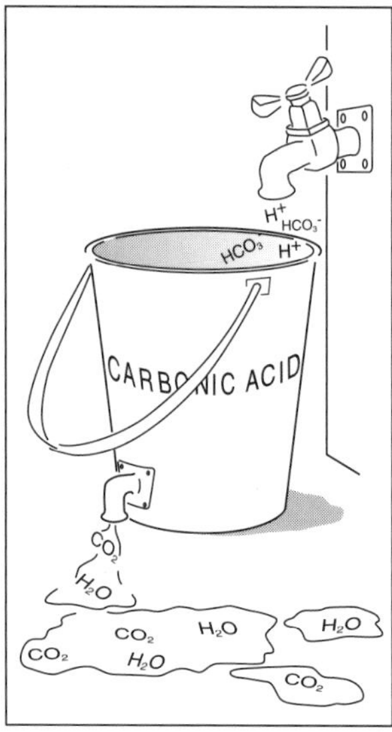

Figure 2.12 Cartoon—showing that carbonic acid preferentially forms carbon dioxide rather than hydrogen and bicarbonate ions.

very few of these molecules are available to break down into hydrogen and bicarbonate ions (figure 2.12). Saturation cannot therefore occur because overall there is little movement of the reaction to the left.

Halt: Key point

Saturation of the carbonic acid-bicarbonate buffer does not occur because carbonic acid is continuously breaking down into carbon dioxide and water

Though the carbonic acid-bicarbonate buffer system is not restricted by saturation, it is limited by the initial concentration of bicarbonate. If this is low to start off with there would be less bicarbonate available to react with the hydrogen ions and so less carbonic acid (and ultimately, therefore, less carbon dioxide and water) is formed. As a result more of the extra hydrogen ions would remain free (that is, "unbuffered") in the extracellular fluid, and the patient would be acidotic.

Standard and actual bicarbonate

A common base found in the body is bicarbonate (HCO_3^-). As will be described in chapter 3, its concentration in the blood depends on both the respiratory and metabolic components of the acid-base balance. There are therefore two measures of bicarbonate.

Standard bicarbonate is the concentration of bicarbonate in a sample of plasma kept under precise "standard" conditions (that is, 37°C and $PaCO_2$ of 40 mm Hg or 5·3 kPa). These particular conditions are chosen to eliminate the changes in bicarbonate resulting from respiration. This needs to be carried out when you want to assess the metabolic components of the acid-base balance. In a normal person the standard bicarbonate has a range of 21–27 mmol/l.

Halt: Key points

- **A standard bicarbonate above 27 mmol/l indicates a metabolic alkalosis**
- **A standard bicarbonate below 21 mmol/l indicates a metabolic acidosis**

As mentioned previously there are several types of buffers in the extracellular fluid. Considering the "standard" conditions mentioned in the previous paragraph you will see that they take into account only the carbonic acid-bicarbonate system. Consequently the "standard bicarbonate" underestimates the metabolic changes because it does not measure how active the other buffers (for example, plasma proteins) have been in trying to maintain the pH in the normal range.

Actual bicarbonate is the concentration of bicarbonate measured in a sample of plasma without the corrections mentioned above. Consequently, the actual bicarbonate reflects the contributions of both the respiratory and metabolic components of the body's acid-base balance. It therefore does not accurately assess the metabolic component in isolation. A common example of an actual bicarbonate measurement is the bicarbonate concentration measured in a venous blood sample. This has a normal range of 21–28 mmol/l.

Base excess and base deficit

These assess how much excessive base or acid is in the blood as a result of a defect in the metabolic system. This is calculated by measuring the amount of strong acid (or base) that has to be added to a sample of blood to produce a pH of 7·4 under the specified conditions stated for "standard bicarbonate". Base excess and deficit take into account all the buffers in the blood sample and are therefore considered a more accurate assessment of the metabolic component of the patient's acid-base status.

It follows therefore that a base excess of 3 mmol/l means that 3 mmol of a strong acid had to be added to each litre of the original sample to get the pH to 7·4 while it was kept at 37°C and a $PaCO_2$ of 40 mm Hg (5·3 kPa). Conversely, a base deficit of 3 mmol/l means that 3 mmol of a strong base had to be added to each litre of the original sample to get the pH to 7·4 while it was kept under the same conditions mentioned above.

To simplify the report form, many laboratories use only the term "base excess".* In these cases a base deficit is described as a negative base excess. With the above examples a "base deficit" of 3 mmol/l would be written as −3 mmol/l and the true "base excess" of 3 mmol/l would be written as +3 mmol/l. The normal range of values for a base excess described in this way is ±2·0 mmol-l (figure 2.13).†

Halt: Key points

- **A base excess below −2·0 mmol/l indicates a metabolic acidosis**
- **A base excess above +2·0 mmol/l indicates a metabolic alkalosis**

* This may help the laboratories but it has done nothing to help doctors and nurses trying to understand acid-base!

† For those who are interested some blood gas analysers call the base excess the "actual base excess" and use the label "ABE" on the printouts. This is to distinguish it from the standard base excess (SBE), which takes into account variation in the buffering ability of different parts of the body's extracellular fluid. Though the SBE is normally −3 to +3 mmol/l, there is no advantage in practice by using it rather than the ABE.

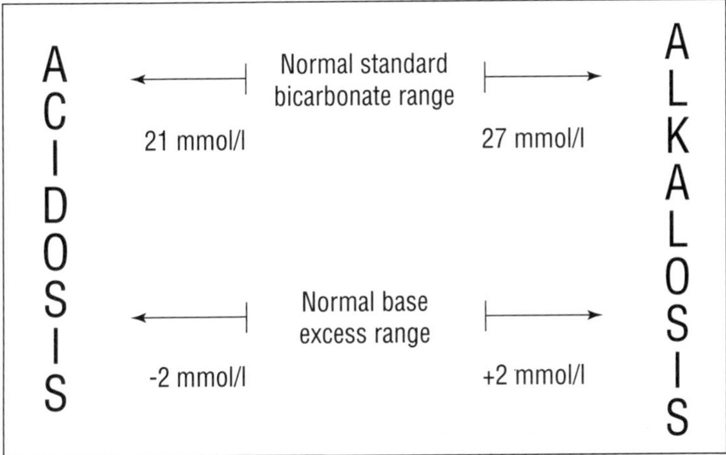

Figure 2.13

Ventilation and respiration

Though these terms are often used interchangeably, they do refer to two separate processes. In this book we define these as:

- Ventilation is the movement of gas into and out of the lungs (that is, the pre-alveolar movement)
- Respiration is the chemical process occurring at a cellular level whereby oxygen is used up to produce energy and carbon dioxide is produced as a waste product.

Summary

There are certain basic terms used in discussing acid-base problems. If you can answer correctly all the questions in quiz 2 then you can be assured that you have these terms mastered. If you miss out on a few don't panic, just take the opportunity to read this chapter again and have another go. You may also find it helpful to read the next few chapters and keep referring back to the appropriate section of this chapter.

Quiz

This chapter has discussed the main terminology you will come across in this book. Go and make yourself a cup of coffee and think for a few minutes about what you have read. When you come back take the opportunity to test your comprehension by having a go at quiz 2 below.

Quiz 2 (answers on page 150–2)

1 **How many grams of sodium chloride are there in 10 ml of a 1 molar solution?**
2 **How much lignocaine (lidocaine) is there in 10 ml of a 2% solution?**
3 **What is the partial pressure of carbon dioxide in dry air at sea level?**
4 **What is the partial pressure of nitrogen in dry air at sea level?**
5 **What does PaO_2 mean?**
6 **What is 40 mm Hg expressed in kPa?**
7 **What is the difference between an acidaemia and an acidosis?**
8 **What is the difference between a base and an alkali?**
9 **Name an intracellular and extracellular buffer?**
10 **What does a base excess of −6 mmol/l mean?**

3 Acid production and its removal

PETER DRISCOLL

Objectives

- To understand how the body eliminates carbon dioxide
- To understand how the body eliminates the acid produced by metabolism
- To show how these two systems work together.

All of us, whether we are healthy or ill, produce large amounts of water, acids, and carbon dioxide each day (box 3.1). These are the waste products of the food we have metabolised to release energy. As this process occurs at a cellular level it is here that these products initially accumulate and go on to produce irreparable cellular damage if left unchecked.

As described previously the first acute compensatory mechanism is the intracellular buffering system. This provides the cell with a temporary way of minimising the fluctuations in acidity. Subsequently, these waste products (that is, carbon dioxide and hydrogen ions) are excreted into the blood stream where they are taken up by the extracellular buffers (figure 3.1).

If this was the sum total of the body's defence to acids and carbon dioxide, however, then the buffers would soon become saturated, allowing the products of metabolism to accumulate in the blood stream. Buffers therefore represent only a temporary

Box 3.1 Normal acid production

A healthy adult will normally produce the equivalent of about 14 570 000 000 nmol of hydrogen ions each day as part of the waste products of metabolism

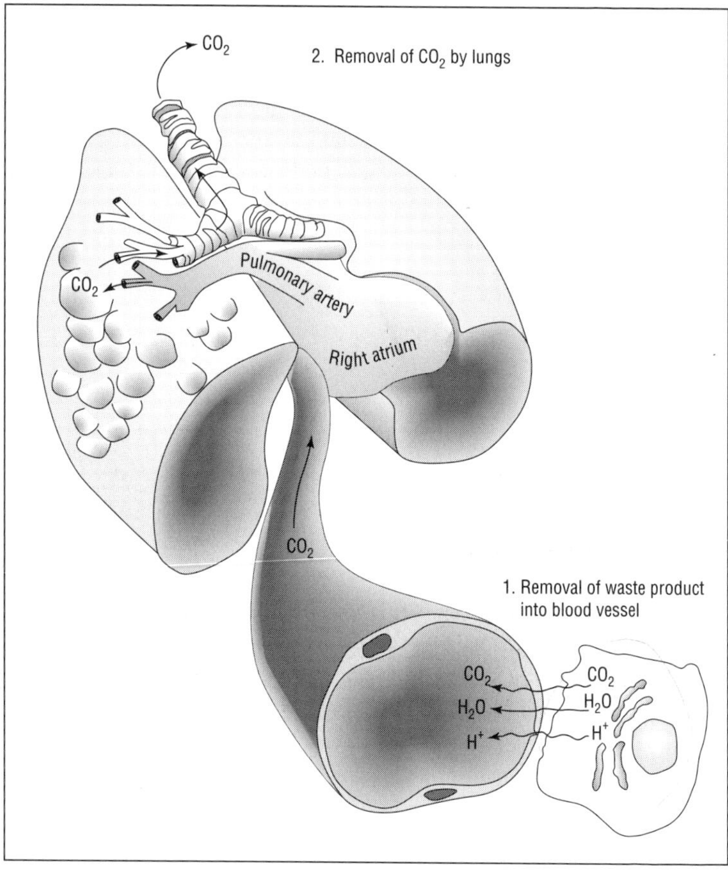

Figure 3.1 Removal of waste products into blood vessel and removal of CO_2 by lungs.

solution. Consequently a system is needed to remove these harmful substances from the body and, at the same time, regenerate the buffers. Fortunately the body has two waste disposal systems to eliminate these toxic byproducts and these represent the two sides of the body's acid-base balance. Let us look at each of these in turn.

Carbon dioxide removal (the respiratory component of the acid base balance)

The carbon dioxide (CO_2) produced by cellular activity is transported in the blood to the lungs. After passing into the alveoli it is removed from the body during expiration (figure 3.1).

Around 5% of the CO_2 transported in the blood is attached to plasma proteins and haemoglobin with a similar amount simply dissolved in intracellular and extracellular fluid. The remaining 90% reacts with water molecules inside and outside the cells to produce hydrogen ions (H^+) and small amounts of bicarbonate (HCO_3^-):

$$\xleftarrow{\qquad\qquad\qquad\qquad\qquad}$$

$$H^+\uparrow + HCO_3^-\uparrow \leftrightarrow H_2CO_3 \leftrightarrow CO_2\uparrow + H_2O$$

> **Halt: Key points**
>
> **When you consider the respiratory component of the body's acid-base balance:**
>
> - **CO_2 should be considered to be an acid because when it dissolves in blood it reacts with water to give H^+**
> - **The greater the amount of CO_2 the more the reaction moves to the left and the more H^+ are produced**

Most blood gas machines will give you a value for the "total carbon dioxide in the patient's plasma (TCO_2)". This is the quantity of carbon dioxide dissolved in plasma plus the plasma bicarbonate concentration. It is normally between 24–28 mmol/l and does not include an approximately equal amount of carbon dioxide contained in the red cells.

A normal person at rest will excrete about the equivalent of 13 000 000 000 nmol of H^+/day through the lungs. It is therefore easy to see that there can be a rapid onset of acidosis should ventilation be compromised for any reason. As the underlying process giving rise to the acid-base disturbance is the result of an abnormality in the respiratory component of the body's acid-base balance, this condition is known as a **respiratory acidosis**.

Should the increase in plasma concentration of hydrogen ions exceed the capacity of the body's buffers then free hydrogen ions will accumulate in the plasma. When the concentration of these free hydrogen ions is large enough to cause the pH to fall below 7·36 a **respiratory acidaemia** will have been produced. If a sample of arterial blood was taken immediately this occurred then the following result would be obtained:

Measure	Normal	Respiratory acidaemia
pH	7·36–7·44	⇊
$PaCO_2$	35–45 mm Hg (4·7–6·0 kPa)	↑
Actual HCO_3^-	21–28 mmol/l	↑
Standard HCO_3^-	21–27 mmol/l	21–27 mmol/l
Base excess	±2 mmol/l	±2 mmol/l

As mentioned above the reaction between carbon dioxide and water leads to more bicarbonate being produced. This is measured as a small increase in the actual bicarbonate concentration.* In contrast, the standard bicarbonate and base excess remain unchanged because these depend on the metabolic components of the body's acid-base balance.

Halt: Key points

- **An increase in carbon dioxide changes the concentration of hydrogen ions sufficient to cause the pH to change**
- **There is a rise in the concentration of actual bicarbonate**
- **The concentration of standard bicarbonate and base excess remain constant**

Acid removal (the metabolic component of the acid-base balance)

Daily cellular metabolism gives rise to about 1 570 000 000 nmol of H^+.† This acid load is subsequently soaked up by buffers in the blood stream so that they can be transported

* Can you remember the difference between actual and standard bicarbonate? Check your answer with page 33.)

† An important source of these hydrogen ions is the oxidation of sulphur containing amino acids in ingested proteins.

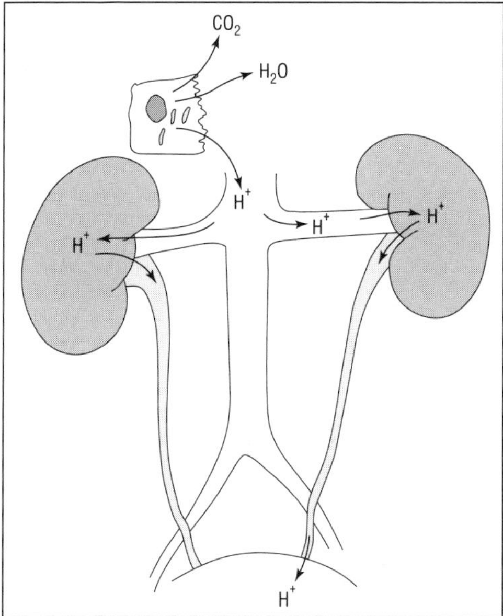

Figure 3.2 Hydrogen ion removal into blood vessel and excreted by kidney.

safely to their point of elimination, which is mainly in the urine (figure 3.2).

A very important buffer is the carbonic acid-bicarbonate system. This generates HCO_3^-, which reacts with the free hydrogen ions released by the cells. As a result there is normally a small fall in HCO_3^- concentration. The kidneys are a substantial source of bicarbonate used in this manner but other organs, such as the gut and liver, also contribute (figure 3.3).

Halt: Key point

The result of a metabolic acid load is a fall in the bicarbonate concentration

If the capacity of all the extracellular fluid buffers is exceeded there will be an accumulation of free hydrogen ions in the plasma. As the process giving rise to the acid-base disturbance is a result of an abnormality in the metabolic component of the body's acid-base

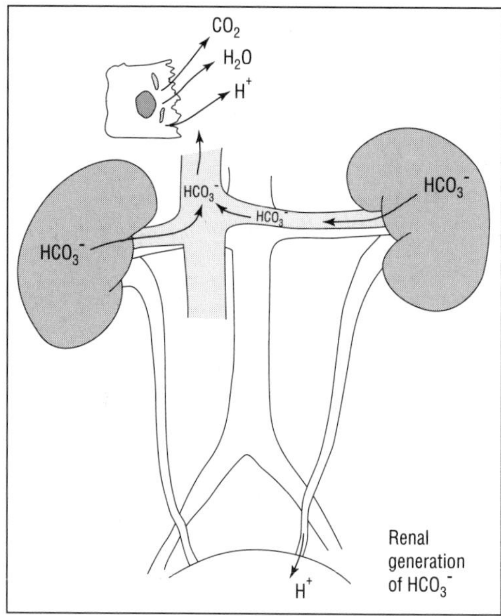

Figure 3.3 Bicarbonate production by the kidney.

balance, this condition is known as a metabolic acidosis.* Should sufficient hydrogen ions be produced to cause the pH to fall below 7·36 then the term **metabolic acidaemia** would be used to describe the patient's condition.

If the breathing was kept constant in a patient with metabolic acidaemia the following results would be obtained from a sample of his or her arterial blood:

Measure	Normal	Metabolic acidaemia
pH	7·36–7·44	↓↓
$PaCO_2$	35–45 mm Hg (4·7–6·0 kPa)	↑
Actual bicarbonate	21–28 mmol/l	↓
Standard HCO_3^-	21–27 mmol/l	↓
Base excess	±2 mmol/l	↓

The increase in carbon dioxide is very small because it is by the same amount as the increase in free hydrogen ions concentration—that is, in the order of nmol/l. As the actual bicarbonate is affected

* The term "metabolic" is used because several organs other than the kidneys are involved in providing bicarbonate ions. It is also called "non-respiratory" by some authors. These people would therefore write "non-respiratory acidosis" when referring to "metabolic acidosis".

by both the respiratory and metabolic components of the body's acid-base balance it falls in this situation because the standard bicarbonate concentration has fallen.

Halt: Key points

- **CO_2 and acids are being produced continually by cell metabolism**
- **The body has two methods of removing these waste products of metabolism and thereby maintaining acid-base balance**
- **The removal of CO_2 by the lungs is the respiratory component of the body's acid-base balance**
- **The production of bicarbonate and excretion of hydrogen ions by the kidney is the main part of the metabolic component of the body's acid-base balance**

The respiratory-metabolic link

It can be seen from the above that the body has two distinct methods of preventing the accumulation of hydrogen ions and the subsequent development of an acidosis. As a further protection against the accumulation of these waste products these two disposal systems are linked so that each can compensate for a derangement in the other.

This link between the respiratory and metabolic systems is due to the presence of **carbonic acid** (H_2CO_3) (figure 3.4).* The association between the hydrogen and bicarbonate ions occurs very quickly, but the breakdown of carbonic acid to carbon dioxide and water normally happens very slowly. This reaction can be speeded up considerably, however, by the enzyme called carbonic anhydrase (also known as carbonic dehydratase).† As this is present in abundance in red cells and kidneys it is ideally placed to facilitate the link between the respiratory and the metabolic systems.

As a result of this link, defects in the metabolic component of the body's acid-base balance can be compensated for by alterations in the amount of carbon dioxide expired. Similarly the link will also

* Do you recognise this link? It is none other than the carbonic acid-bicarbonate buffer system described on page 28.
† In fact it goes about 13 000 times faster!

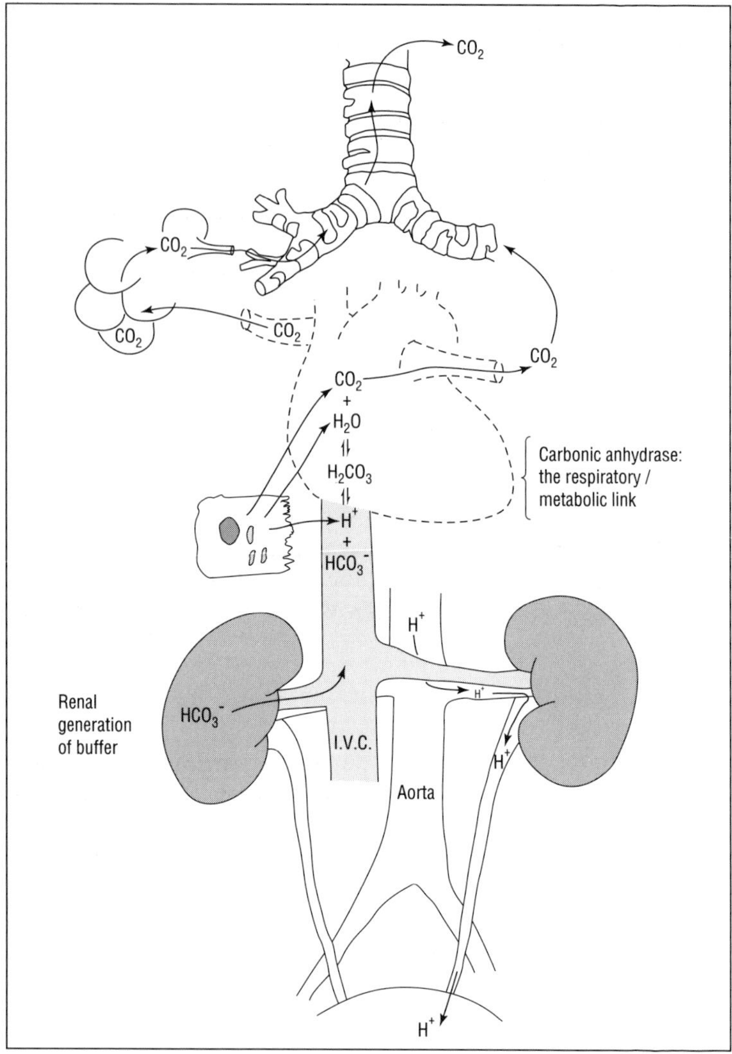

Figure 3.4 Waste product transfer into blood vessel, CO_2 removal by lungs. Hydrogen ion excreted by kidney with bicarbonate production.

allow a defect in the respiratory component to be compensated for by the kidneys altering the amount of hydrogen ions passed in the urine and bicarbonate ions produced by the kidneys. We will discover in chapters 5 and 6 that this link is used when the body has to deal with either too much acid or too much base.

Tip: a way of picturing this is to imagine that:

- **When there is too much metabolic acid, the excess is converted (by the link) into a respiratory acid (that is, carbon dioxide) and removed by the lungs**
- **When there is too much respiratory acid, the excess is converted (by the link) into a metabolic acid (that is, hydrogen ions) and removed mainly by the kidneys**

Summary

With regard to acid-base balance the body keeps the pH within a tight range so that normal cellular metabolic function can continue. The balance depends on the removal of carbon dioxide (the respiratory component of the acid base balance) and the removal of acid (the metabolic component of the acid-base balance). These systems are linked by the carbonic acid-bicarbonate buffer, which enables one system to compensate for a defect in the other.

Quiz

This chapter has discussed how the body normally deals with the acid it produces each day. Go and produce a few acids by having a sandwich and think for a few minutes about what you have read. When you come back take the opportunity to test your comprehension by having a go at quiz 3 below.

Quiz 3 (answers on page 152):

1. **Is acid production abnormal?**
2. **What is the body's first line of defence against an acid load?**
3. **What are the normal arterial partial pressure ranges of CO_2 in a person breathing room air?**
4. **What is the normal plasma pH range and what does this represent in nmol of H^+/l?**
5. **What is the standard bicarbonate range in an arterial blood sample taken from a normal person breathing room air?**
6. **What happens to the concentrations of H^+ and actual**

HCO_3^- in extracellular fluid when carbon dioxide is released into it?

7 **What happens to the concentration of standard HCO_3^- in extracellular fluid when H^+ is released into it?**

8 **Where is carbonic anhydrase found in large amounts in the body?**

9 **How does the respiratory component of the acid-base balance compensate for a metabolic defect?**

10 **How does the metabolic component of the acid-base balance compensate for a respiratory defect?**

4 Understanding oxygenation

CARL GWINNUTT, PETER DRISCOLL

Objectives

- To describe how oxygen is taken up by the lungs and delivered to tissues of the body
- To discuss the differences between the saturation and partial pressure of oxygen.

Oxygen cascade

For tissues to survive, oxygen has to be delivered to them from the atmosphere. This is achieved by the respiratory and cardiovascular systems working together so that the following sequence of events can take place:

- Oxygen delivery to the lungs
- Transfer of oxygen into the blood
- Oxygen carriage by the blood
- Oxygen delivery to the tissues
- Release of oxygen to the tissues.

A break at any point in this sequence will lead to a deficiency in tissue oxygenation, and this is called hypoxia.

Oxygen will pass from the atmosphere, to blood, to tissues, only if in doing so it moves from a relatively high "concentration". You will remember from chapter 2 that when we refer to mixtures of gases the term partial pressure is used rather than concentration. Consequently there is a gradual fall in the partial pressure of oxygen in the different phases of the sequence (table 4.1). This is referred to as the oxygen cascade (figure 4.1).

You will see from table 4.1 that there is a drop of almost one

Table 4.1 The oxygen cascade

Mean partial pressure of oxygen	Inspired air	Trachea	Alveolar gas	Arterial blood	Peripheral tissues
mm Hg (kPa)	159 (21·2)	149·5 (19·9)	109·6 (14·6)	100 (13·3)	25 (3·3)

third in the partial pressure of oxygen between the atmosphere and the alveoli. There are several reasons for this.

Firstly, when atmospheric air is drawn into the lungs it becomes saturated with water vapour. As water vapour has a partial pressure

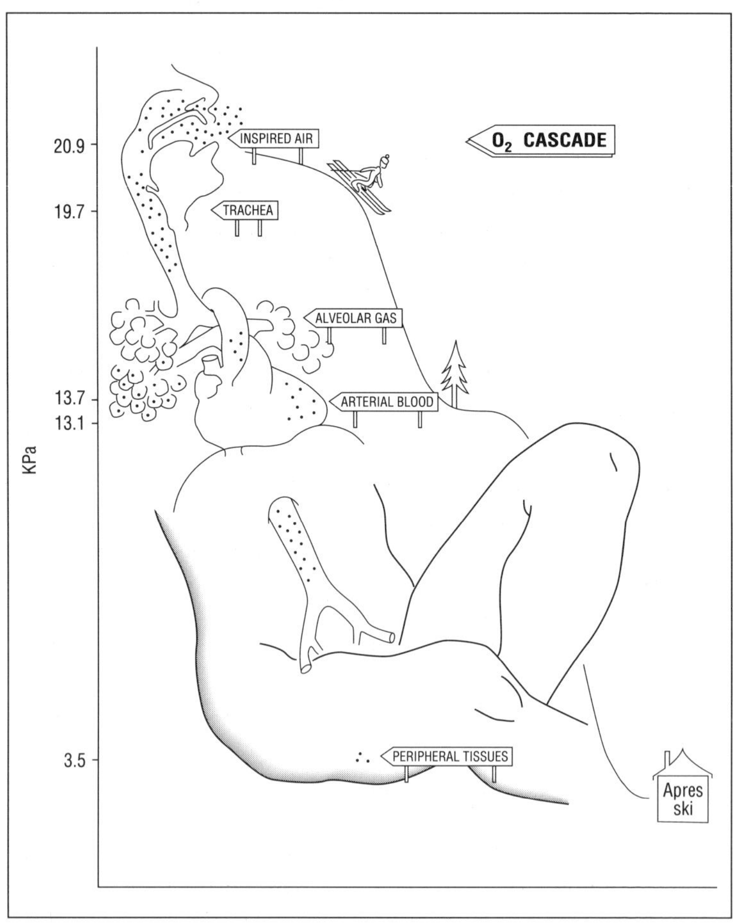

Figure 4.1 Oxygen cascade.

of 47 mm Hg (6·3 kPa), the partial pressure of oxygen changes from:

$$\text{in air} = \%\ \text{volume} \times \text{atmospheric pressure}$$
$$= 20{\cdot}98/100 \times 760\ \text{mm Hg}$$
$$= 159\ \text{mm Hg}\ (21{\cdot}2\ \text{kPa})$$

to:

$$\text{in the trachea} = \%\ \text{volume} \times (\text{atmospheric pressure} - \text{water vapour pressure})$$
$$= 20{\cdot}98/100 \times (760 - 47)\ \text{mm Hg}$$
$$= 149{\cdot}5\ \text{mm Hg}\ (19{\cdot}9\ \text{kPa}).$$

Secondly, alveolar gas also contains about 40 mm Hg (5·3 kPa) of CO_2, which has been delivered to it from the body tissues. This further reduces the space available in the alveoli for oxygen.

Thirdly, and very importantly, there is a continual uptake of alveolar oxygen by the blood and replacement by the arrival of fresh gas (figure 4.2).

Halt: Key points

The fall in the partial pressure of oxygen is because:

- **The addition of water vapour and carbon dioxide to the gas in the alveoli will reduce the partial pressure of oxygen already present because the total partial pressure of all the gases must still equal 760 mm Hg (101 kPa)**
- **Oxygen is continuously diffusing out of the alveoli into the surrounding capillaries**

The amount of oxygen reaching the lungs

From what has been said above it is not surprising that the amount of oxygen reaching the lungs depends on both the partial pressure of oxygen in the inspired gas and the amount of gas reaching the alveoli. We will consider each in turn.

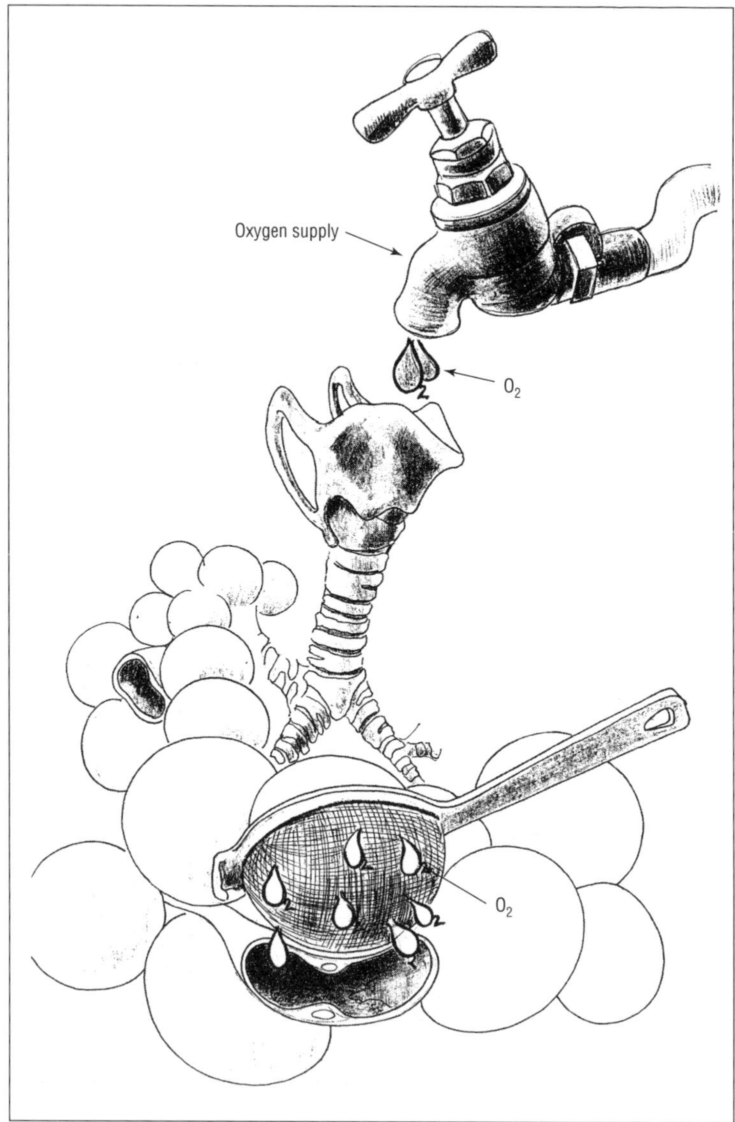

Figure 4.2 The alveolar wall acts like a sieve. There is a continuous leak of oxygen through the alveolar wall into the surrounding blood vessel.

The partial pressure of oxygen in the inspired gas

Increasing or decreasing the amount of oxygen in the inspired gas causes the alveolar partial pressure to change in the same direction but not necessarily by the same amounts. Consider what happens to the PAO_2 when the inspired gas is changed from room air to 40% oxygen:

$$PAO_2 = [\% \text{ volume} \times (\text{atmospheric pressure} - \text{water vapour pressure})]$$

$$- \text{pressure of carbon dioxide in the alveoli}$$

Therefore the PAO_2 with inspired room air:

$$= [20{\cdot}98/100 \times (760 - 47)] - 40 = 109{\cdot}6 \text{ mm Hg } (14{\cdot}6 \text{ kPa})$$

and the PAO_2 with an inspired oxygen concentration of 40%:

$$= [40/100 \times (760 - 47)] - 40 = 245{\cdot}2 \text{ mm Hg } (32{\cdot}7 \text{ kPa})$$

Compare this increase to the fall in PAO_2 that occurs when the inspired oxygen concentration is reduced to 15%:

$$= [15/100 \times (760 - 47)] - 40 = 67 \text{ mm Hg } (8{\cdot}9 \text{ kPa}).$$

This example demonstrates that by almost doubling the percentage of inspired oxygen to 40% we have more than doubled the normal PAO_2. In contrast, by reducing the percentage of inspired oxygen by only a quarter to 15% we have almost halved the PAO_2 (figure 4.3). The reason for this disproportionate effect is because the partial pressure of carbon dioxide and saturated vapour pressure in the alveoli remain the same.

Halt: Key point

The fall in PAO_2 after a reduction in the concentration of inspired oxygen is greater than the rise in PAO_2 after the same increase in the concentration of inspired oxygen

Alveolar ventilation

The process of moving air into and out of the lungs is called **ventilation**. The amount of inspired air that reaches the alveoli and is available for gas exchange is called the **alveolar ventilation**. When the rate and depth of ventilation are reduced (a condition known as **hypoventilation**), less oxygen is delivered per minute to the alveoli to replace that which has been taken up by the blood. This causes the partial pressure of oxygen within the alveoli to fall. As mentioned above, this can be compensated for by increasing the concentration of oxygen in the inspired gas. If ventilation continues to fall, however, a point will eventually be reached when compensation is no longer possible. For any subsequent reduction in inspired concentration the PAO_2 will fall precipitously.

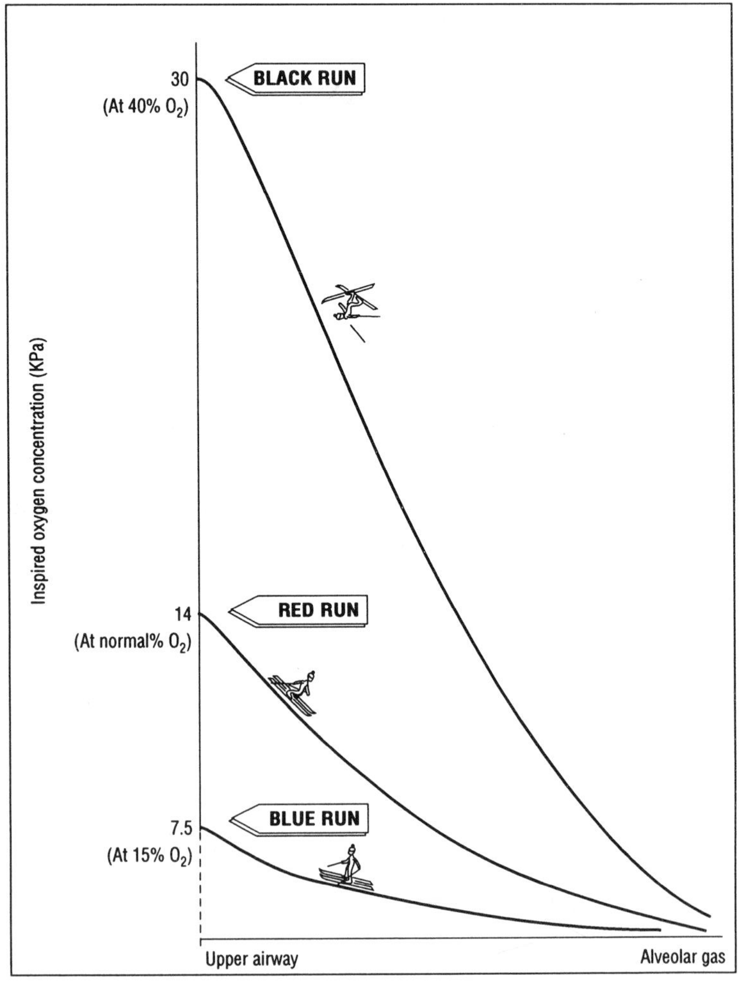

Figure 4.3 A reduction in inspired oxygen produces a marked fall in PAO_2.

Halt: Key point

Hypoventilation always reduces PAO_2 unless there is an increase in the inspired oxygen concentration sufficient to compensate

Transfer of oxygen into the blood

In the alveoli, gases are separated from the blood by a thin membrane. Movement across this is termed **diffusion**, and the rate at which this occurs is affected mainly by the following factors (figure 4.4).

- The surface area of the membrane separating the gas and blood
- The thickness of the membrane
- The difference in partial pressure of the gas across the membrane
- The solubility of the gas in blood.*

The structure of the lung is ideally suited for the transfer of gases either from the alveoli to the blood (for example, oxygen) or from the blood to the alveoli (for example, carbon dioxide). The total surface area of the membrane is about the size of a tennis court (about 100 m^2) and is very thin (0·0005 mm). The difference in partial pressure for oxygen between alveoli and arterial blood, however, is about 10 mm Hg (1·3 kPa) under normal circumstances.

The rate of diffusion is also proportional to the solubility of a gas.† Compared with other gases in the body, such as carbon dioxide, oxygen is not particularly soluble. The dimensions of the membrane mentioned above, however, more than compensate for this. Consequently, under normal circumstances the combination of all the factors affecting transfer will enable the red blood cells in the pulmonary capillaries to collect their maximum limit of oxygen in less than 0·25 second. As the time taken by red cells to travel along the pulmonary capillaries is about 0·75 second in resting

* For those who like lists, the diffusion of gases across the alveolar membrane also depends on the size of the molecules in the gas and the solubility of the gas in the fluid lining the alveoli. These factors, however, have a much smaller effect compared with those above.

† Solubility depends on the temperature of the gas and its partial pressure. Interestingly an increase in temperature usually results in a decrease in solubility.

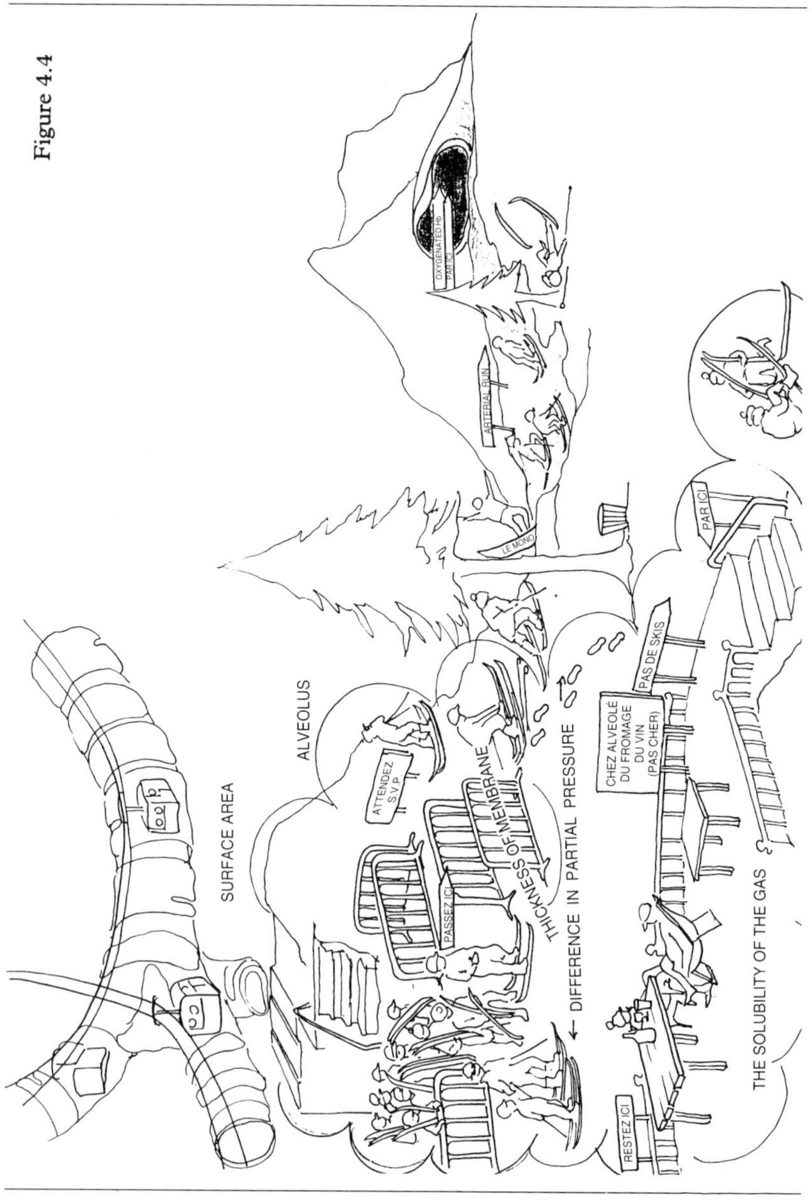
OXYGENATED Hb
PAR ICI
ARTERIAL RUN
LE MONO
PAR ICI
PAS DE SKIS
CHEZ ALVEOLÉ
DU FROMAGE
DU VIN
(PAS CHER)
ALVEOLUS
SURFACE AREA
ATTENDEZ
S.V.P.
THICKNESS OF MEMBRANE
PASSEZ ICI
← DIFFERENCE IN PARTIAL PRESSURE →
THE SOLUBILITY OF THE GAS
RESTEZ ICI

Figure 4.4

healthy people, there is also normally a great deal of diffusion reserves.

Oxygen carriage by the blood

Haemoglobin

If the oxygen carrying ability of blood relied only on how much could be dissolved in plasma our tissues would not survive. The reason being that only 0·3 ml of oxygen dissolves in every 100 ml of blood in a patient breathing room air.* With a normal cardiac output of 5000 ml/min this would result in the delivery of 15 ml O_2 per minute to the tissues (that is, $5000 \times 0{\cdot}3/100$). As the normal resting demand for oxygen is 250 ml/min, this is clearly inadequate. Therefore a system is needed to increase the oxygen carrying capacity of blood so that the delivery of oxygen to the tissues can be improved.

This extra help is provided by the presence of haemoglobin,

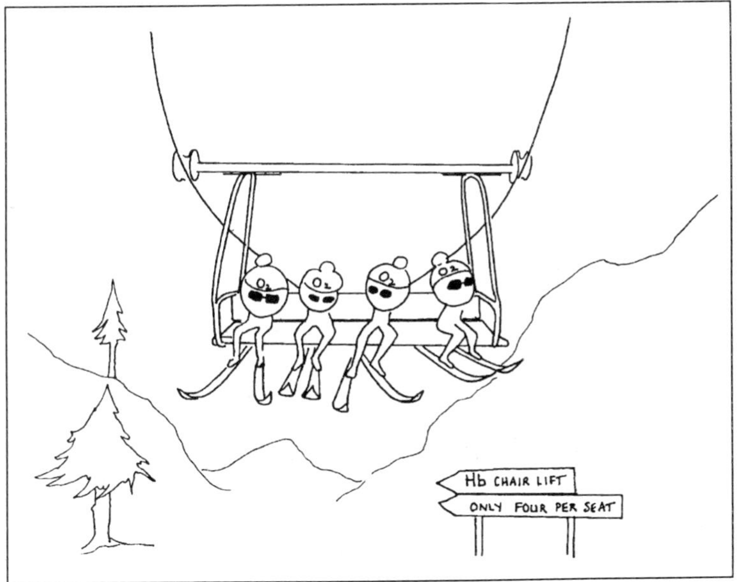

Figure 4.5

* This is assuming that the person is at sea level—that is, the atmospheric pressure is 760 mm Hg (101 kPa). If a patient was on top of a mountain this pressure would be less and so would the amount of oxygen dissolved in the plasma.

which is contained within the red blood cells at an average concentration of 15 g per 100 ml of blood. Each molecule of haemoglobin can carry four molecules of oxygen (figure 4.5).

When haemoglobin is fully saturated with oxygen it is called oxygenated haemoglobin or **oxyhaemoglobin** and when deoxygenated it is called **deoxyhaemoglobin**. When deoxyhaemoglobin is exposed to oxygen, the uptake of each molecule of oxygen facilitates the uptake of the remainder.† This process occurs in less than 0·01 seconds and is called association. The opposite of this — that is, the off loading of oxygen—is known as dissociation (figure 4.6).

Once all the haemoglobin molecules have taken up 4 oxygen molecules, the haemoglobin is said to be 100% saturated. This is often expressed as $SaO_2 = 100\%$, where S = saturation and a = arterial.

When the $SaO_2 = 100\%$, each gram of haemoglobin in the arterial system is carrying 1·34 ml oxygen—a figure known as the oxygen carrying capacity of haemoglobin. Consequently each

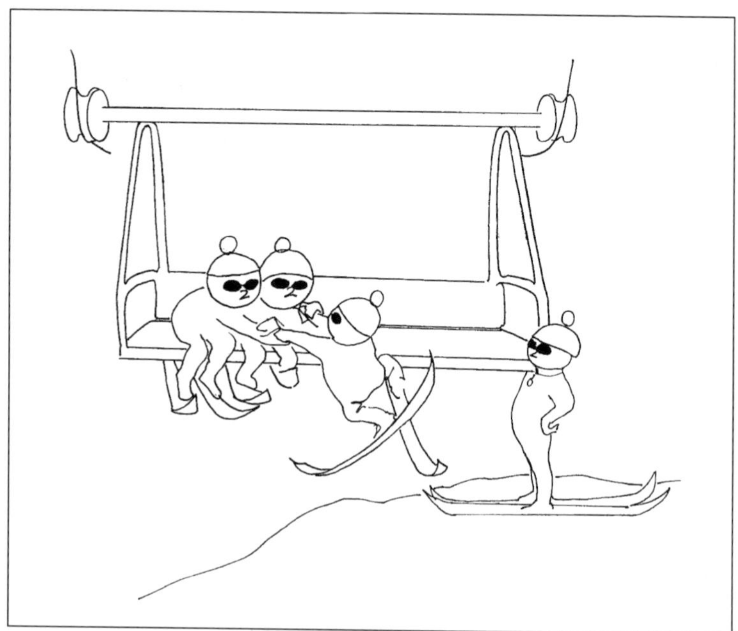

Figure 4.6 Oxygen molecules give a helping hand.

† For those readers who are interested, this property is known as the quaternary function of haemoglobin.

100 ml of arterial blood, containing 15 g haemoglobin, will carry $15 \times 1 \cdot 34 = 20 \cdot 1$ ml oxygen. Compare this to the 0·3 ml of oxygen that would be carried if the oxygen was merely dissolved in the blood.

> **Halt: Key point**
>
> **The presence of haemoglobin allows about 60 times more oxygen to be carried than would be possible if blood relied simply on oxygen dissolved in the plasma**

A saturation of 100%, however, is achieved only if haemoglobin is exposed to a PAO_2 of 250 mm Hg. If it is exposed to a lower partial pressure then it will be less than fully saturated. This can be represented graphically to produce a curve (figure 4.7). The rapid uptake of oxygen is represented by the initial steep slope of the curve, where small changes in PaO_2 cause large changes in the saturation. Beyond a PAO_2 of 50–60 mm Hg the curve becomes flatter as little further saturation occurs despite increases in PAO_2. In the normal situation the PaO_2 is about 100 mg Hg, and this results in a saturation of around 97%.

This curve is called the **oxyhaemoglobin dissociation** curve,

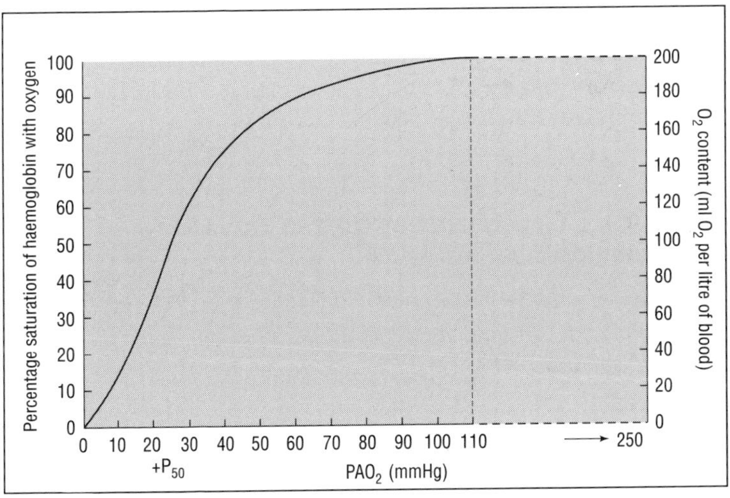

Figure 4.7 Oxyhaemoglobin dissociation curve.

although it clearly relates also to the association of oxygen with haemoglobin.

Figure 4.7 shows that the partial pressure of oxygen has to fall considerably before there is any notable change in the saturation reading. Indeed the PaO_2 could fall from 250 mm Hg to 90 mm Hg and the SaO_2 would change only from 100% to about 97%. Below 90 mm Hg, however, the fall gets steeper, indicating there is a large drop in SaO_2 for every mm Hg fall in PaO_2.*

The oxygen content of blood

Although most oxygen is carried in the blood by haemoglobin, we have also mentioned that an additional small volume is physically dissolved in plasma. Therefore the total volume of oxygen carried in blood at any time is the sum of that carried by the haemoglobin (box 4.1) plus that dissolved in the plasma. This total is termed the **oxygen content.**

The volume of oxygen dissolved in plasma from arterial blood is directly proportional to the PaO_2 and is about:

$$0{\cdot}003 \text{ ml per 100 ml blood per mm Hg } PaO_2$$

or

$$0{\cdot}023 \text{ ml per 100 ml blood per kPa } PaO_2$$

It follows that the oxygen content per 100 ml of arterial blood (that is, the amount associated with the haemoglobin molecule (Hb) as well as that dissolved in the plasma) is equal to:

> **Box 4.1 The volume of oxygen carried by haemoglobin depends on**
>
> - The haemoglobin concentration in the blood
> - The oxygen carrying capacity of the haemoglobin
> - The saturation of haemoglobin with oxygen

* This has implications on how you should interpret the readings from pulse oximeters, which are often used in clinical practice to measure the saturation of oxygen.

(Hb conc $\times$ oxygen carrying capacity of Hb saturation of Hb) oxygen content of haemoglobin $+ (0{\cdot}003 \times PaO_2)$ oxygen content of the plasma

which is:

$$\text{Hb conc} \times 1{\cdot}34 \times \text{saturation of Hb}) \quad + (0{\cdot}003 \times PaO_2)$$

For simplicity we have just used the values for PaO_2 measured in mm Hg. For those using kPa you will need to alter the equation in the way indicated on page 21.

Consider now a normal person who has a PaO_2 of 100 mm Hg with a haemoglobin concentration of 15 g per 100 ml that is 97% saturated with oxygen. In this person the oxygen content per 100 ml of arterial blood would be equal to:

$$(15 \times 1{\cdot}34 \times 97\%) + (0{\cdot}003 \times 100)$$

$$= 19{\cdot}5 + 0{\cdot}3$$

$$= 19{\cdot}8 \text{ ml oxygen per 100 ml blood}$$

Now consider two situations. In the first, the inspired oxygen concentration is increased such that the PaO_2 is 400 mm Hg. This will result in the haemoglobin being 100% saturated. In this case the oxygen content per 100 ml blood will be:

$$(15 \times 1{\cdot}34 \times 100\%) + (0{\cdot}003 \times 400)$$

$$= 20{\cdot}1 + 1{\cdot}2$$

$$= 21{\cdot}3 \text{ ml oxygen per 100 ml blood}$$

In the second example, the PaO_2 is reduced to 30 mm Hg, resulting in the haemoglobin being 57% saturated. In this case the oxygen content per 100 ml blood will be:

$$(15 \times 1{\cdot}34 \times 57\%) + (0{\cdot}003 \times 30)$$

$$= 11{\cdot}5 + 0{\cdot}09$$

$$= 11{\cdot}6 \text{ ml oxygen per 100 ml blood}$$

Halt: Key points

- **Increasing the PaO_2 above 100 mm Hg has its major effect on increasing the volume of oxygen dissolved in the plasma**
- **Decreasing the PaO_2 leads mainly to a reduction in the volume of oxygen carried by haemoglobin**
- **Even at a low PaO_2 there is still a considerable amount of oxygen in the blood that can act as an oxygen reserve**

Oxygen delivery to the tissues

So far we have considered only the volume of oxygen in terms of how much oxygen is contained in aliquots of 100 ml of blood when it is exposed to varying partial pressures of oxygen. Under normal circumstances the heart is pumping out 5000 ml blood per minute (the cardiac output). Therefore the total volume of oxygen delivered to the tissues per minute is the product of the cardiac output and the oxygen content:

$$\text{oxygen delivery } (DO_2) = \text{cardiac output} \times \text{oxygen content}$$

$$\text{in normal circumstances } DO_2 = 5000 \text{ ml/min} \times 19{\cdot}8 \text{ ml/100 ml}$$

$$= \text{about } 1000 \text{ ml oxygen/min}$$

This value will clearly be affected by changes in the cardiac output and oxygen content, either separately or in combination. In practice, however, increases in oxygen delivery are achieved mainly by increasing the cardiac output (for example, during exercise) because the potential for further increases in the oxygen content is small. As we have seen in the previous example, this is the case even if the inspired concentration is increased considerably.

Larger effects on the delivery of oxygen can occur if either value falls—for example, there is a reduction in the amount of oxygen that could be carried by each litre of blood in patients with a low haemoglobin concentration. Although this would cause the DO_2 to fall, the reduction would be limited by the body increasing the cardiac output as a means of compensation. A life threatening fall in oxygen delivery, however, can occur when both the cardiac output and the oxygen capacity are reduced. An example of this is seen in trauma victims who have lost over 30% of their blood volume (around 1·5–2 litres in an average adult). In this situation the cardiac output falls because there is less blood in the circulation. Furthermore, there is also less haemoglobin to carry oxygen to the tissues after the trauma. As a result, less blood is delivered to the tissues per minute and what is delivered is carrying less oxygen. This rapidly leads to hypoxia, anaerobic metabolism.*

Release of oxygen to the tissues

The partial pressure gradient

When arterial blood arrives at the tissues it enters an environment where the partial pressure of oxygen is much lower. Consequently, despite the affinity of haemoglobin for oxygen there is movement of oxygen molecules from haemoglobin through the plasma and into the tissues down the partial pressure gradient (figure 4.8). Under normal circumstances, however, not all of the oxygen is removed from the blood passing through the tissues. For example, at rest the body's requirement for oxygen is about 250 ml a minute. As the total volume of oxygen available at any time is 1000 ml, however, only 25% of the available oxygen is removed from the haemoglobin. Therefore venous blood is still 75% saturated, even though the partial pressure of oxygen has fallen to just 40 mm Hg. This represents another reserve that allows the body to adapt to conditions when the oxygen demand is increased—for example, during exercise or illness.

The oxygen content of venous blood can be calculated as follows:

$$= (\text{Hb} \times 1{\cdot}34 \times \text{oxygen saturation of venous blood}) + (0{\cdot}003 \times \text{PvO}_2)$$

$$= (15 \times 1{\cdot}34 \times 75) + (0{\cdot}003 \times 40)$$

$$= 15{\cdot}08 + 0{\cdot}12$$

$$= 15{\cdot}2 \text{ ml oxygen/100 ml blood}$$

Other factors affecting the release of oxygen at the tissues

The release of oxygen from haemoglobin to the tissues is facilitated by the steep lower part of the haemoglobin dissociation curve (see figure 4.7). This enables large amounts of oxygen to be released from the blood for only a small drop in the partial pressure

* Anaerobic metabolism occurs when food is broken down without the benefit of oxygen. As a result less energy and more acids are produced, and tissue damage.

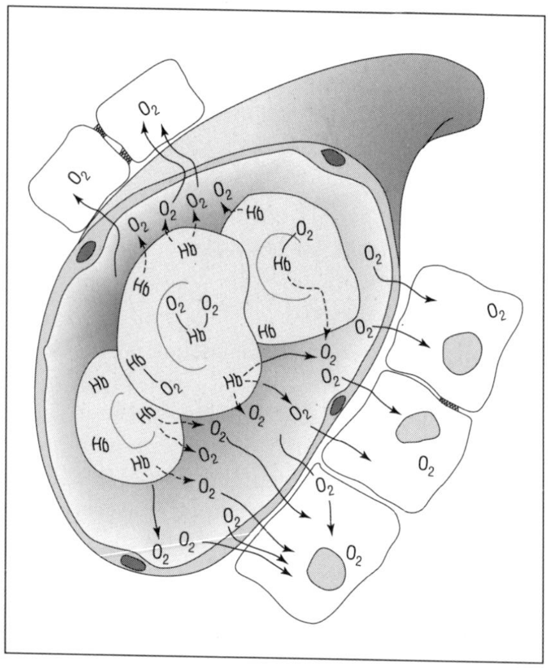

Figure 4.8 Movement of oxygen from Hb in red blood cells into plasma in the blood vessels and then into tissues, proceeding in the direction of partial pressure gradient.

of oxygen in the capillaries.

Various local factors can also affect the ability (or affinity) of the haemoglobin molecules to carry oxygen while they circulate in the capillaries perfusing the tissues. The most important of these factors is the acidosis in the tissues as a result of their metabolic activity. This local fall in the pH has the effect of "shifting" the haemoglobin dissociation curve to the right of its position in figure 4.7—that is, for a given saturation the PaO_2 is greater (figure 4.9). This means that more oxygen is released in close proximity to the tissues that require it. The same effect is seen with increases in temperature and partial pressure of CO_2. The shift in the oxygen dissociation curve as a result of changes in $PaCO_2$ is known as the Bohr effect. As active muscles exhibit all these features, the delivery of oxygen to them is greatly assisted.

An indication of the amount of shift of the oxygen dissociation curve can be gained from checking the P_{50}. This is the partial pressure of oxygen required to saturate 50% of the haemoglobin

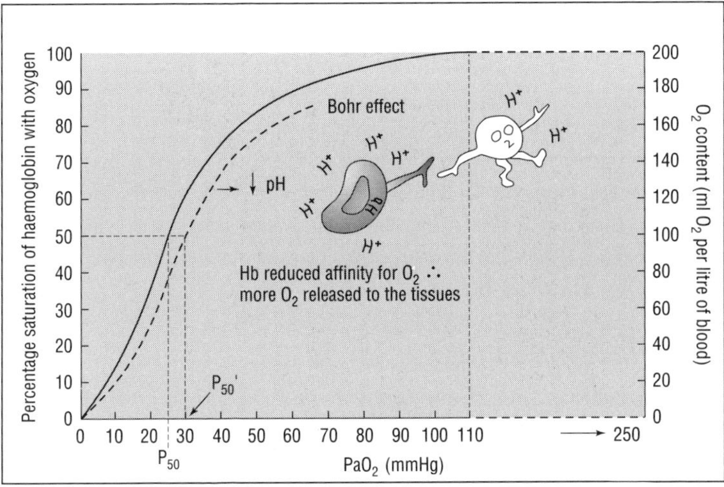

Figure 4.9 A shift in the oxyhaemoglobin dissociation curve to the right course an increase in P_{50}.

(figure 4.9). It is normally around 27 mm Hg (3·6 kPa) and is often provided with the blood gas result.

Halt: Key points

- **A rise in $PaCO_2$, hydrogen ions, and temperature shifts the haemoglobin dissociation curve to the right**
- **A rise in the P_{50} indicates a shift in the haemoglobin dissociation curve to the right**
- **A fall in the P_{50} indicates a shift in the haemoglobin dissociation curve to the left**

Summary

A partial pressure gradient for oxygen is an important factor in the movement of oxygen between the atmosphere and the tissues. Furthermore, oxygen transportation from the lungs to the tissues by the blood is greatly facilitated by the presence of haemoglobin. This increases the carrying capacity 60–70-fold. In comparison oxygen dissolved in the plasma plays only a very minor role.

PaO_2 is normally sufficient to saturate haemoglobin almost fully with oxygen. Furthermore, under normal cirumstances the delivery of oxygen to the tissues greatly exceeds demand and as a result there is usually a considerable reserve of oxygen in the blood.

Quiz

This chapter has discussed many of the fundamental factors that affect oxygen delivery to the body's tissues. Make yourself a cup of tea and think for a few minutes about what you have read. When you come back take the opportunity to test your comprehension by having a go at quiz 4 below.

Quiz 4 (answers on page 152–4)

1 **Name the stages the oxygen molecule has to go through to get from the atmosphere to the tissues?**
2 **Why is the partial pressure of oxygen lower in the alveoli compared with the atmosphere?**
3 **What factors affect the rate of diffusion of oxygen across the alveoli membrane?**
4 **What is the oxygen capacity of haemoglobin?**
5 **What is the mean partial pressure of oxygen in arterial blood?**
6 **What is the relation between the oxygen saturation of blood and the partial pressure of oxygen?**
7 **What is the oxygen content of a blood sample from a patient who has an oxygen saturation of 97%, a haemoglobin concentration of 15 g/100 ml, and a PaO_2 of 85 mm Hg?**
8 **Why does a decrease, as opposed to an increase, in PaO_2 have a bigger effect on the oxygen content of arterial blood?**
9 **What is the oxygen delivery in the patient in question 7 if his or her cardiac output was 4 l/min?**
10 **Name three factors that cause the oxygen dissociation curve to be shifted to the right?**

5 Common acidoses

PETER DRISCOLL

Objectives

- To discuss the mechanisms and causes of common respiratory and metabolic acidoses
- To describe how the body compensates for these acidotic states
- To discuss what happens when there is a combined respiratory and metabolic acidosis
- To provide clinical examples of these types of acid-base disturbances.

Respiratory acidosis

The oxygen in the alveoli is replenished by the process of moving air into and out of the lungs (ventilation). Therefore if we multiplied the volume of air breathed in (that is, the tidal volume) by the number of breaths per minute (that is, the respiratory rate) then we would arrive at a figure known as the minute ventilation. This is the amount of gas inhaled each minute and in normal adults this amounts to:

$$\text{minute ventilation} = 500 \text{ ml} \times 15 = 7{\cdot}5 \text{ l/min}$$

Not all the inhaled gas reaches the alveoli, some has to remain in the proximal airways (figure 5.1). In fact with a normal tidal volume of 500 ml, only 350 ml (70%) gets to the alveoli.* You will remember from chapter 4 (page 51) that this volume is called the alveolar ventilation and represents the amount of the inhaled air that is available to undergo exchange with gases in the pulmonary capillaries (figure 5.2).

It follows that if **alveolar ventilation** is reduced, less carbon dioxide can be removed from the body. This retention will lead in turn to a rise in $PaCO_2$ (**hypercapnia**) and produce a respiratory acidosis.

* The tidal volume is normally equal to 7–8 ml/kg.

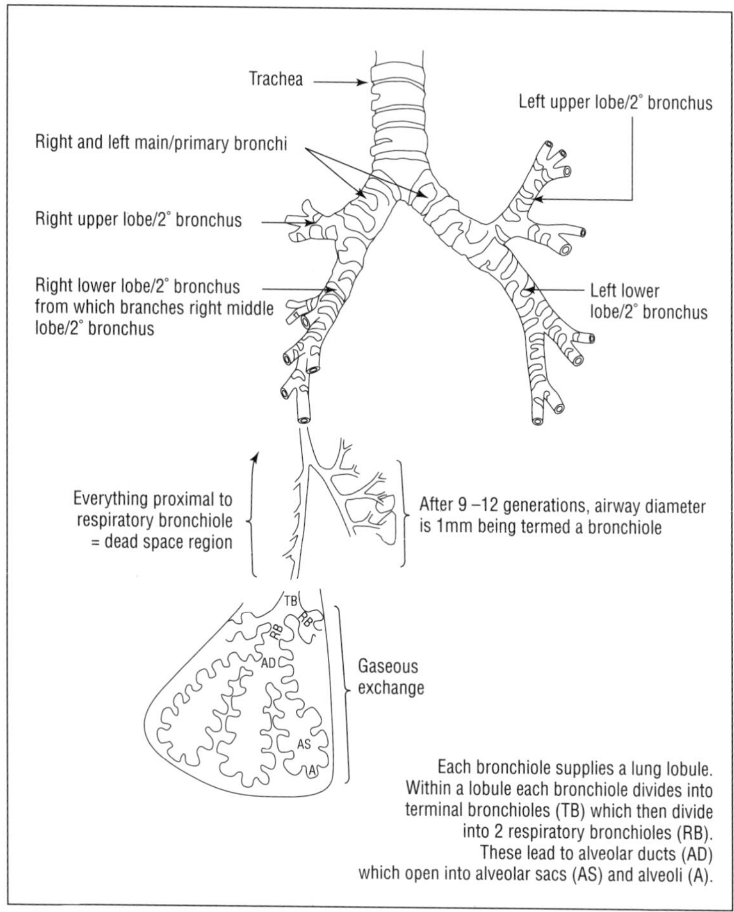

Figure 5.1 Airways anatomically marked plus alveoli and dead space region.

Acute respiratory acidosis

There are several causes for an acute respiratory acidosis, but the most common is inadequate alveolar ventilation (box 5.1).

The accumulation of carbon dioxide in extracellular fluid enables more CO_2 to react with water molecules to produce hydrogen ions:

$$\xleftarrow{\hspace{6cm}}$$

$$H^+\uparrow + HCO_3^-\uparrow \leftrightarrow H_2CO_3 \leftrightarrow CO_2\uparrow + H_2O$$

Box 5.1 Common causes of acute respiratory acidosis

- Upper airway obstruction—for example, foreign body
- Lower airway obstruction—for example, severe asthma
- Impaired alveolar filling—for example, bronchopneumonia
- Depression of the respiratory centre—for example, drugs

If a sample of arterial blood was taken in the acute situation then the following result would be obtained:

Measure	Normal	Respiratory acidaemia
pH	7·36–7·44	↓↓
$PaCO_2$	35–45 mm Hg (4·7–6·0 kPa)	↑
Actual HCO_3^-	21–28 mmol/l	↑
Standard HCO_3^-	21–27 mmol/l	21–27 mmol/l
Base excess	±2 mmol/l	±2 mmol/l

The actual bicarbonate concentration increases as a byproduct of

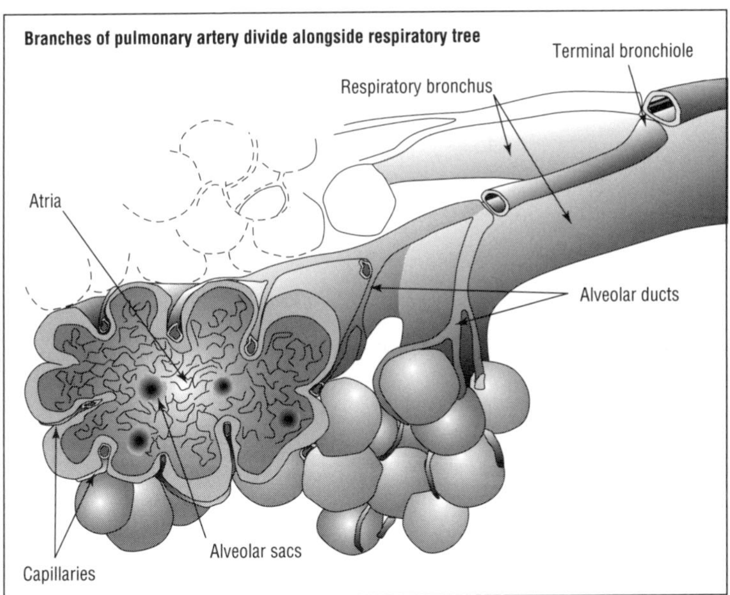

Figure 5.2 Alveoli with neighbouring capillaries.

the reaction between carbon dioxide and water but the amount is usually small—that is, in the order of 1–2 mmol/l. In this early stage there are no metabolic effects on the bicarbonate concentration—consequently the standard bicarbonate and base excess remain constant (confused?—see pages 33 and 34).

Within seconds the blood buffers will start acting on the extra free hydrogen ions. In addition the kidneys can provide extra help by means of the respiratory metabolic link. By exchanging hydrogen ions for bicarbonate the kidneys can prevent bicarbonate being lost in the urine. Consequently they not only help to remove some of the acid load but also provide further bicarbonate to react with the additional free hydrogen ions. As this help is coming from the metabolic component of the body's acid-base balance it is known as **metabolic compensation** (Figure 5.3). Remember this compensation is called "metabolic" rather than simply "renal" because there are similar effects going on in the gut as well. Nevertheless, the kidney is the most important.

Often the initial acid-base disturbance is known as the primary acid-base disturbance to help to distinguish it from the alterations that result from metabolic or respiratory compensation. Therefore by using the above situation, you could call this a primary respiratory acidosis with metabolic compensation.

It is important to realise that although the renal mechanism comes into play immediately, it takes 2–5 days to build up sufficient HCO_3^- throughout the body. This delay in achieving maximum efficiency would be extended even further if the severity of the respiratory acidosis gradually increased rather than remaining constant.

If a sample of arterial blood was taken once metabolic compensation had taken effect then the following result would be obtained:

Measure	Normal	Respiratory acidaemia	Metabolic compensation
pH	7·36–7·44	↓↓	↓
$PaCO_2$	34–45 mm Hg (4·7–6·0 kPa)	↑	↑
Actual HCO_3^-	21–28 mmol/l	↑	↑↑
Standard HCO_3^-	21–27 mmol/l	21–27 mmol/l	↑
Base excess	±2 mmol/l	±2 mmol/l	↑

The metabolic compensation is reflected in the rise of standard

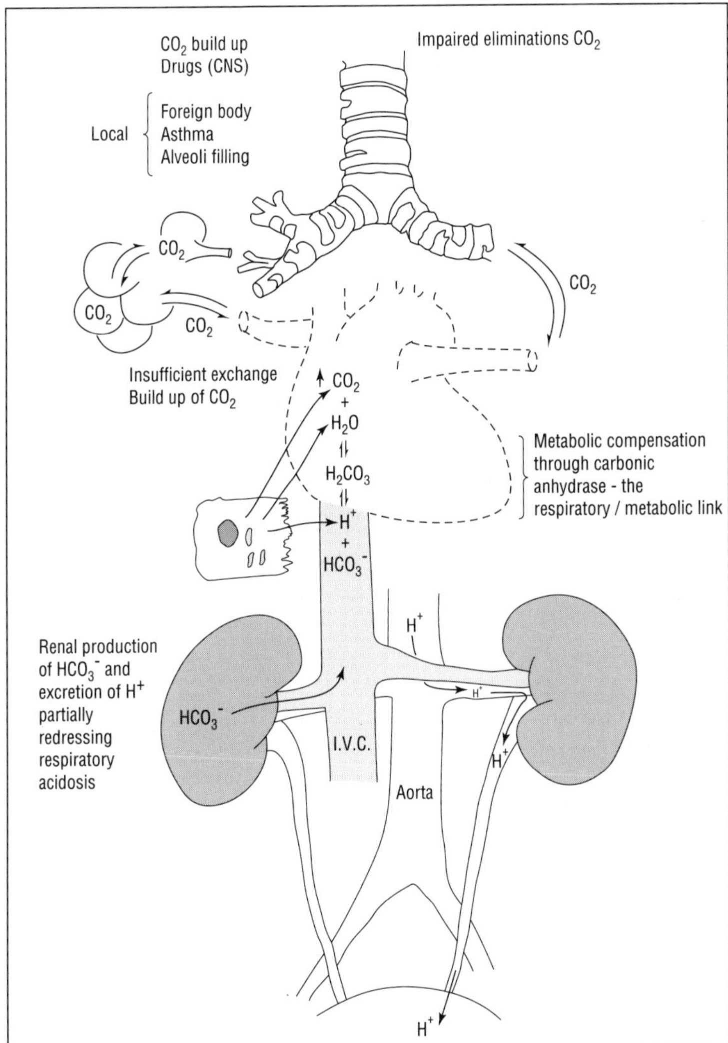

Figure 5.3 Acute respiratory acidosis and metabolic compensation.

bicarbonate concentration and base excess. Furthermore, this increase in standard bicarbonate causes the actual bicarbonate concentration to increase by a similar amount.

Usually in these acute situations there is only a small rise in the standard bicarbonate and base excess concentrations. Consequently, the body does not overcompensate and an acidaemia (that is, low pH) remains. Nevertheless, the pH is nearer to the normal range than it was before the compensation. How close it gets to normality depends on the severity of the primary respiratory acidosis and the degree of compensation. You will also notice from these results that the $PaCO_2$ is constant, indicating that in this case the severity of the underlying respiratory acidosis is unchanged.

Halt: Key points

- **Compensation means that the abnormal hydrogen ion concentration is brought back towards normal; usually acute compensation is not complete, and the pH will remain outside the normal range**
- **Compensation does not mean the restoration of normal blood chemistry; there would still be clear abnormalities in the $PaCO_2$, standard bicarbonate, and base excess concentration.**

Figure 5.4 depicts these changes for those who like to use graphs.

Halt: Key points

- **Respiratory acidosis is associated with a rise in $PaCO_2$**
- **The metabolic component of the body's acid-base balance can compensate for a respiratory acidosis by increasing the elimination of hydrogen ions and increasing bicarbonate concentration**
- **Metabolic compensation usually takes 2–5 days to achieve an optimal level**

To put these changes into context it is best to review some real life clinical examples.

Example 1

History—A 19 year old man was deposited in the emergency department by his colleagues 5 minutes after injecting heroin. He had shallow respiration at a rate of 7/min, and he responded only to painful stimuli.

Results—While the patient was breathing 85% oxygen via a non-rebreathing mask with reservoir, an arterial sample was taken for blood gas analysis. The results were:

Measure	Normal	Patient
pH	7·36–4·44	7·2
$PaCO_2$	35–45 mm Hg (4·7–6·0 kPa)	71 mm Hg (9·5 kPa)
Actual HCO_3^-	21–28 mmol/l	26·5 mmol/l
Standard HCO_3^-	21–27 mmol/l	26·0 mmol/l
Base excess	±2 mmol/l	− 1·4 mmol/l

Analysis—The patient's history indicates that there has probably been depression of the respiratory centre after the heroin injection.

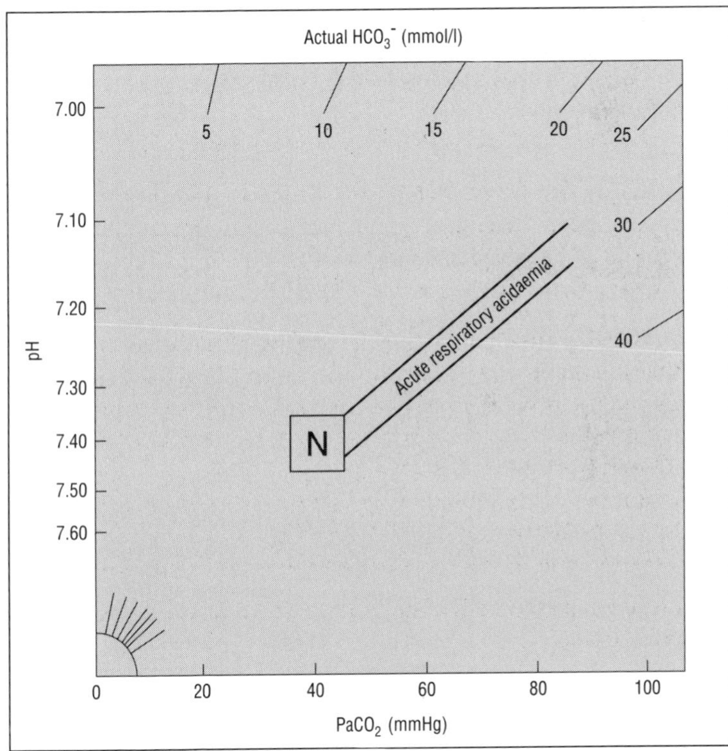

Figure 5.4 This graph shows how pH alters with changes in $PaCO_2$. The diagonal lines indicate the concentration of actual bicarbonate. The square box N indicates the normal range for pH, $PaCO_2$ and actual bicarbonate concentration. Fanning out from this box is the possible range of values associated with an acute respiratory acidaemia.

From a clinical point of view, therefore, it would be reasonable to suspect that this patient could have developed a respiratory acidosis.

Do the results support this clinical proposal? The answer to this is yes because:

- The pH is low, indicating there is an acidaemia
- The $PaCO_2$ is high, indicating there is a respiratory acidosis
- The standard bicarbonate and base excess are within the normal range.

Putting these all together you can conclude that this patient has developed a respiratory acidosis after an injection of heroin. The rise in $PaCO_2$ has produced enough free hydrogen ions to cause the pH to fall (that is, an acidaemia has been produced). We can see that there has been insufficient time to develop metabolic compensation because the standard bicarbonate and base excess are within the normal range.

Example 2

History—A six year old girl was brought into the emergency department after having a grand mal convulsion at home. Her parents had given her rectal diazepam, and the fit had resolved. On arrival in the department she was drowsy but rousable.

Results—While the patient was breathing 30% oxygen via mask, an arterial sample was taken for blood gas analysis. The results were:

Measure	Normal	Patient
pH	7·36–7·44	7·31
$PaCO_2$	34–45 mm Hg (4·7–6·0 kPa)	56·7 mm Hg (7·6 kPa)
Actual HCO_3^-	21–28 mmol/l	28·0 mmol/l
Standard HCO_3^-	21–27 mmol/l	27·0 mmol/l
Base excess	±2 mmol/l	+2·0 mmol/l

Analysis—The patient was drowsy and may have had depressed respiration as a result of the diazepam. If this were the case, we would expect to see a respiratory acidosis as a consequence of the inadequate ventilation allowing the $PaCO_2$ to rise.

Do the results support this clinical proposal? The answer to this is yes because:

- The pH is low, indicating that there is an acidaemia
- The $PaCO_2$ is high, indicating there is a respiratory acidosis
- The standard bicarbonate and base excess are at the upper limit of normal.

Putting these all together it is likely that this patient has developed a respiratory acidosis secondary to hypoventilation. This has produced enough free hydrogen ions to cause an acidaemia. Furthermore, the high normal values for standard bicarbonate and base excess indicates that the process has been going on long enough for the body to start to develop some metabolic compensation.

Chronic respiratory acidosis

If the cause of the respiratory acidosis is long standing (box 5.2) the body will be able to develop metabolic compensation that keeps pace with the extra acid load. Consequently, you do not see the uncompensated picture typical of acute respiratory acidosis. Instead the patient's pH is normal or nearly normal, depending on whether the compensation is complete or not. In either case, however, the $PaCO_2$ and HCO_3^- concentration will be abnormally high in chronic respiratory acidosis.*

Figure 5.5 depicts these changes for those who like to use graphs.

The following clinical example also helps to demonstrate these changes.

Example 3

History—A 67 year old woman was admitted to hospital for a total hip replacement. She was known to be suffering from COPD but was currently well controlled. As part of her routine preoperative assessment an arterial blood gas analysis was carried out.

Box 5.2 Common causes of chronic respiratory acidosis

- Lower airway obstruction—for example, chronic obstructive pulmonary disease (COPD), emphysema
- Impaired alveolar filling—for example, kyphoscoliosis

* Look back to pages 25–6, if the pH was normal (that is, there was full compensation) but the $PaCO_2$ and bicarbonate concentration increased, then there would be a respiratory acidosis but no acidaemia.

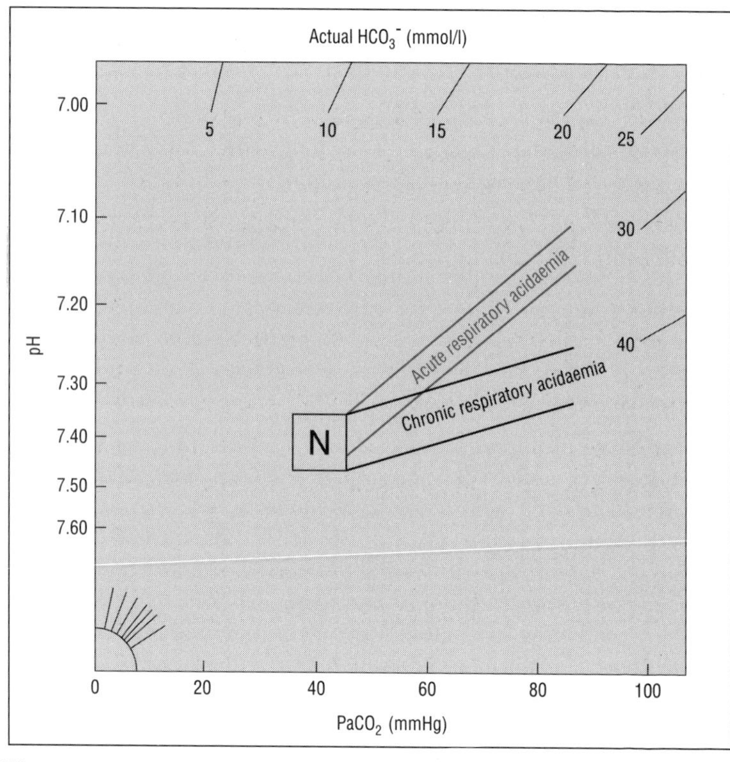

Figure 5.5 The possible ranges associated with chronic respiratory acidaemia, superimposed on figure 5.4.

Results—While the patient was breathing room air an arterial sample was taken for blood gas analysis. The results were:

Measure	Normal	Patient
pH	7·36–7·44	7·35
$PaCO_2$	35–45 mm Hg (4·7–6·0 kPa)	60 mm Hg (8·0 kPa)
Actual HCO_3^-	21–28 mmol/l	32·0 mmol/l
Standard HCO_3^-	21–27 mmol/l	30·0 mmol/l
Base excess	±2 mmol/l	+4 mmol/l

Analysis—Respiratory acidosis occurs in patients with inadequate alveolar ventilation—for example, chronic bronchitis—because of the accumulation of carbon dioxide. Over time, however, the metabolic system compensates by increasing bicarbonate production by the kidneys. We would therefore expect such a result in this patient.

Do the results support this proposal? The answer is yes, because:

- The pH is slightly low, indicating a mild acidaemia
- The $PaCO_2$ is high, indicating a respiratory acidosis
- The standard bicarbonate and base excess are raised.

The small reduction in pH indicates that the degree of metabolic compensation is almost complete.

Example 4

History—A 60 year old woman with an inoperable carcinoma of the bronchus was brought into the emergency department complaining of increasing shortness of breath and drowsiness.

Results—While the patient was breathing room air an arterial sample was taken for blood gas analysis. The results were:

Measure	Normal	Patient
pH	7·36–7·44	7·33
$PaCO_2$	35–45 mm Hg (4·7–6·0 kPa)	70·4 mm Hg (9·4 kPa)
Actual HCO_3^-	21–28 mmol/l	36·5 mmol/l
Standard HCO_3^-	21–27 mmol/l	36·2 mmol/l
Base excess	±2 mmol/2	+7·4 mmol/l

Analysis—As this patient has a condition that can compromise alveolar ventilation she might be retaining carbon dioxide. Such a condition would have been present for some time, however, and so we would expect to see some evidence of metabolic compensation.

The results support this because:

- The pH is low, indicating an acidaemia
- The $PaCO_2$ is raised, indicating a respiratory acidosis
- The standard bicarbonate and base excess are raised.

It is interesting to note here that though there are large alterations in the concentrations of $PaCO_2$, standard bicarbonate, and base excess, the pH is close to normal. This indicates that there has been an almost complete metabolic compensation for the severe respiratory acidosis.

Unfortunately, while in the emergency department the patient rapidly deteriorated and became unresponsive. A repeat arterial sample was taken, which showed:

Measure	Normal	Patient
pH	7·36–7·44	7·17
$PaCO_2$	35–45 mm Hg (4·7–6·0 kPa)	109·8 mm Hg (14·6 kPa)
Actual HCO_3^-	21–28 mmol/l	39·3 mmol/l
Standard HCO_3^-	21–27 mmol/l	39·2 mmol/l
Base excess	±2 mmol/l	+7·6 mmol/l

Here you can see that as alveolar ventilation became worse more carbon dioxide was retained, worsening the acidaemia. Though the metabolic system would normally attempt to compensate by increasing the amount of bicarbonate, it has not had enough time to adapt to the rapid increase in carbon dioxide.

Metabolic acidosis

This condition usually results from an abnormally large acid load. Less commonly it is due to either the loss of bicarbonate or the kidneys being unable to excrete the normal acid load produced by metabolism (box 5.3).

Box 5.3 Causes of metabolic acidosis

Increased H^+ load

- Increased production of hydrogen ions—for example,
  - Lactic acidosis
  - Diabetic ketoacidosis
- Ingestion of hydrogen ions or substances that are metabolised to hydrogen ions—for example,
  - Methanol
  - Alcohol overdose
  - Ethylene glycol

Increased HCO_3^- loss

- Gastrointestinal loss—for example,
  - Diarrhoea
  - Intestinal fistula
- Increased loss from the kidneys—for example,
  - Renal tubular disease
  - Drugs (such as acetazolamide)

Impaired excretion of a normal acid load by the kidneys

Renal failure
Renal tubular disease

Whatever the cause of the metabolic acidosis, there will always be a reduction in the bicarbonate concentration. This important point can be appreciated by considering each of the two possible ways it can occur. If it was due to an excessive acid load then the body's initial response would be to use its buffers. The most important of these is the carbonic acid-bicarbonate system:

$$H^+ + HCO_3^- \leftrightarrow H_2CO_3^- \leftrightarrow CO_2 + H_2O$$

As a result of its reaction with the hydrogen ions, the concentration of bicarbonate would fall. The bicarbonate concentration would also fall if the metabolic acidosis was due to a loss of bicarbonate.

Key point

A metabolic acidosis is always associated with a fall in the bicarbonate concentration

Acute metabolic acidosis

If a sample of arterial blood was taken in this acute situation then the following result would be obtained:

Measure	Normal	Metabolic acidaemia
pH	7·36–7·44	↓↓↓
$PaCO_2$	35–45 mm Hg (4·7–6·0 kPa)	35–45 mm Hg (4·7–6·0 kPa)
Actual HCO_3^-	21–28 mmol/l	↓↓
Standard HCO_3^-	21–27 mmol/l	↓↓
Base excess	±2 mmol/l	↓↓

The reaction between hydrogen ions and bicarbonate will give rise to an increase in the $PaCO_2$. This is by a very small amount because the increase in the hydrogen ion concentration is in the order of several nmol/l. As this very small amount cannot be measured by the blood gas analyser, the $PaCO_2$ appears unchanged.

It is very rare, however, to have a patient with a primary metabolic acidosis that is uncompensated. In practice the rise in hydrogen ions leads to respiratory stimulation within minutes, with maximal compensation within 12–24 hours.* This causes more

* The hydrogen ions are in fact detected by special receptors called chemoreceptors in the carotid and aortic bodies. These then send out impulses that stimulate the respiratory centre located in the brain stem.

carbon dioxide to be eliminated and the $PaCO_2$ to fall. By means of the respiratory-metabolic link (that is, the carbonic acid-bicarbonate buffer system mentioned above) this fall in $PaCO_2$ causes more carbonic acid to break down into carbon dioxide and water. The concentration of carbonic acid therefore falls with the effect that there is even less of it available to break down into hydrogen and bicarbonate ions (see pages 28–32). As a result the direction of the equation is moved further to the right, allowing more of the available bicarbonate to react with the free hydrogen ions (figure 5.6).

Halt: Key point

By means of the carbonic acid-bicarbonate buffer the fall in CO_2 generated by the increase in respiration enables more bicarbonate to react with hydrogen ions

Though the respiratory-metabolic link reduces the actual bicarbonate concentration even further, this fall is small—that is, in the order of mmol/l. In contrast, the fall in the number of hydrogen ions that results from this link has a considerable effect on the pH, returning it towards normal. Consequently, the body can try to counteract the acid load by using this link. As this compensation comes from the respiratory component of the body's acid-base balance it is known as respiratory compensation. It should be remembered also that the degree to which the respiratory system can compensate for a primary metabolic acidosis depends on the work involved in breathing and the systemic effects of a low $PaCO_2$ (hypocarbia).

If a sample of arterial blood was taken once respiratory compensation had occurred the following result would be obtained:

Measure	Normal	Metabolic acidaemia	Respiratory compensation
pH	7·36–7·44	↓↓↓	↓↓
$PaCO_2$	35–45 mm Hg (4·7–6·0 kPa)	35–45 mm Hg (4·7–6·0 kPa)	↓
Actual HCO_3^-	21–28 mmol/l	↓↓	↓↓↓
Standard HCO_3^-	21–27 mmol/l	↓↓	↓↓
Base excess	2 mmol/l	↓↓	↓↓

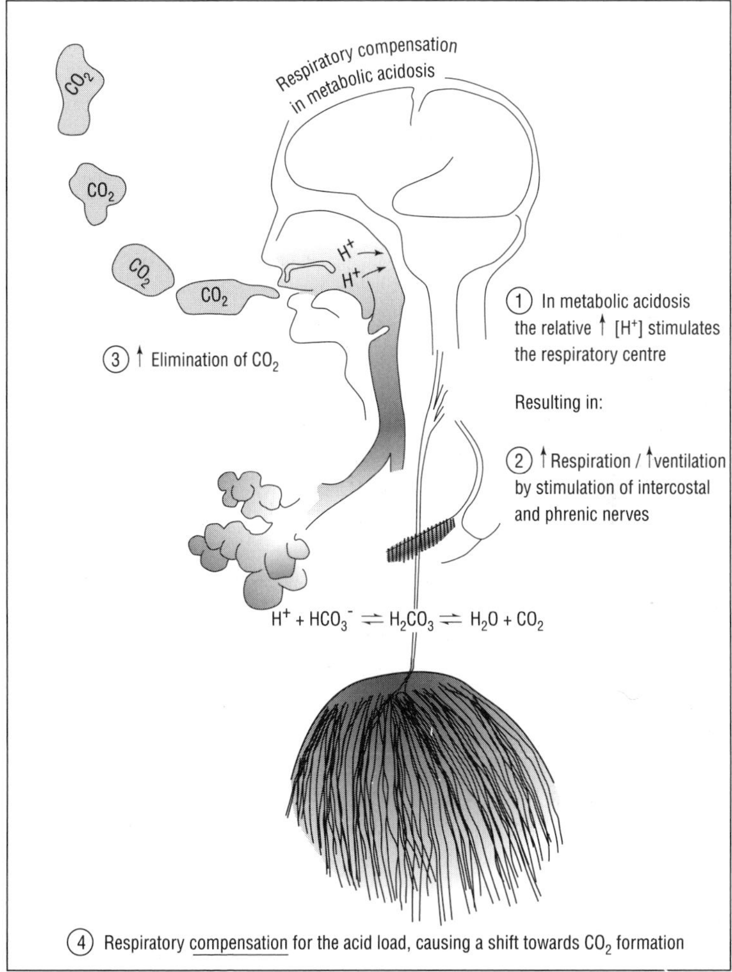

Figure 5.6 Respiratory compensation lowers the CO_2 concentration, therefore allowing more of the available bicarbonate to react with the free hydrogen ions.

In these acute simple situations the body does not overcompensate. Consequently, even though there is a fall in the $PaCO_2$ there is still a persistent acidaemia (that is, low pH). Nevertheless, the pH is nearer to the normal range than it was before the compensation. You will also notice from these results that the actual bicarbonate concentration has fallen further. As described previously, small reductions are in keeping with the respiratory compensation. If the fall in bicarbonate is severe, however, it is more likely that the underlying metabolic acidosis has got worse as well.

Figure 5.7 depicts these changes for those who like to use graphs.

Halt: Key points

- **Metabolic acidosis is associated with a fall in both the standard bicarbonate and base excess concentration**
- **The respiratory component of the body's acid-base balance can compensate for a metabolic acidosis by facilitating the reaction between bicarbonate and hydrogen ions; as a result the actual bicarbonate concentration falls even further**
- **Respiratory compensation usually starts within minutes and is complete within 12–24 hours**
- **Respiratory compensation is limited by the work involved in breathing and the systemic effects of a low $PaCO_2$**

To help put these changes into context, consider the following clinical example.

Example 5

History—A 27 year old epileptic man had a grand mal seizure. The convulsions stopped without medication within a minute after he arrived in the emergency department.

Results—An arterial sample was taken for blood gas analysis soon after the convulsions stopped. At that time the patient was receiving 85% oxygen by a non-rebreathing mask with reservoir. The results were:

Measure	Normal	Patient
pH	7·36–7·44	7·27
$PaCO_2$	35–45 mm Hg (4·7–6·0 kPa)	27·6 mm Hg (3·7 kPa)
Actual HCO_3^-	21–28 mmol/l	12·2 mmol/l
Standard HCO_3^-	21–27 mmol/l	12·9 mmol/l
Base excess	±2 mmol/l	−13·3 mmol/l

Analysis—During convulsions the muscles contract vigorously.

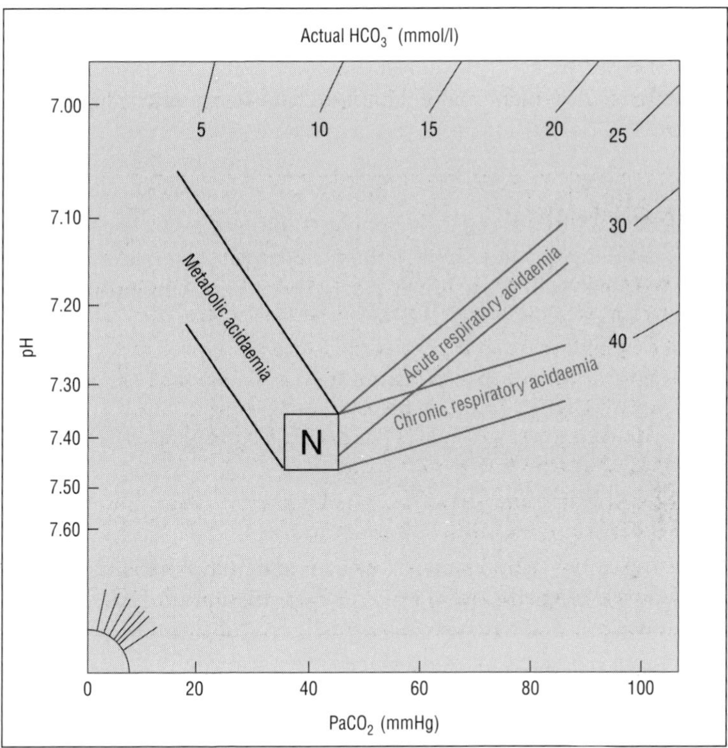

Figure 5.7 Possible ranges associated with metabolic acidaemia, superimposed on figure 5.5.

To gain the extra energy needed to do this they increase their metabolic rate and break down extra amounts of glucose. The amount of oxygen getting to the muscles in this situation, however, is reduced. This is partly because of the contracting muscles causing compression of their blood vessels. A further reason is that generalised convulsions prevent patients from breathing. Therefore, in addition to retaining carbon dioxide (and causing a respiratory acidosis), there is also a reduction in the uptake of oxygen by the lungs. The end result is that the muscles receive less oxygen than they need. The cells of the body cannot simply stop metabolising, however, because they would die. Consequently, those tissues that can change from aerobic (that is, using oxygen) to anaerobic metabolism do so. (Most tissues can make this change, but the notable exceptions are the brain and the heart.) The muscle cells are an example of those tissues that can undergo this change.

Though this allows them to break down some glucose molecules without the need for oxygen, it does produce large quantities of an acid called lactic acid. It follows therefore that during the actual fit the patient has a combined respiratory and metabolic acidosis.

Once the convulsion stops patients usually start breathing and so are able to blow off their retained carbon dioxide. Not only does this correct the respiratory acidosis but also enables respiratory compensation to develop in response to the metabolic acidosis.

From the history therefore one would expect this patient to have developed a metabolic acidosis with respiratory compensation.

Do the results support this clinical proposal? The answer to this is yes because:

- The pH is low, indicating there is an acidaemia
- The standard bicarbonate and base excess are low, indicating there is a metabolic acidosis
- The $PaCO_2$ is low indicating respiratory compensation.

Putting these all together you can conclude that this patient developed a metabolic acidosis after the epileptic fit. Furthermore, this produced enough free hydrogen ions to cause the pH to fall (that is, an acidaemia was produced). We can see that in response the body developed respiratory compensation because the partial pressure of carbon dioxide is below the normal range.

Chronic metabolic acidosis

If the kidney is not the primary cause of the metabolic acidosis then it will be able to help counteract the increased acid load in much the same way that it did in the case of respiratory acidosis. In other words, it is possible to have **metabolic compensation for a metabolic acidosis**. In these circumstances the kidneys excrete more hydrogen ions and prevent bicarbonate being lost in the urine so that there is more HCO_3^- to react with the acid in the body. As the kidney begins to restore the plasma bicarbonate concentration the pH will rise closer to the normal range. Consequently the stimulus to the respiratory centres will fall, allowing the respiratory rate to slow and the $PaCO_2$ to rise slightly.

As described before this metabolic compensation takes 2–5 days to achieve maximum efficiency. If an arterial blood sample was taken once it had come into effect, however, the following result would be obtained:

Measure	Normal	Metabolic acidaemia	Respiratory compensation	Metabolic compensation
pH	7·36–7·44	↓↓↓	↓↓	↓
$PaCO_2$	35–45 mm Hg (4·7–6·0 kPa)	35–45 mm Hg (4·7–6·0 kPa)	↓↓	↓
Actual HCO_3^-	21–28 mmol/l	↓↓	↓↓↓	↓
Standard HCO_3^-	21–27 mmol/l	↓↓	↓↓	↓
Base excess	±2 mmol/l	↓↓	↓↓	↓

Unlike the situation in chronic respiratory acidosis it is rare for the body to be able to compensate fully for a metabolic acidosis, even with the added help from the kidney. Consequently, there is usually a persistent acidaemia (that is, low pH) but the pH will be nearer to the normal range. The $PaCO_2$ as well as the actual and standard concentrations of bicarbonate will also rise slightly as a result of the fall in the respiratory rate and the action of the kidney. Nevertheless, all will remain abnormally low. If the release of acid was gradual, such as found in diabetic ketoacidosis, there would be a slow but continuous transition from one compensation system to another.

To help put these changes into context, consider the following clinical example.

Example 6

History—A 33 year old man with insulin dependent diabetes was brought by helicopter to the emergency department, having been unwell for three days on a wilderness survival course. He initially noticed dysuria and frequency, and quite soon afterwards he developed a pyrexia. Unable to receive medical help he decided to soldier on but over the past 24 hours he had been sweaty, nauseated, and had not been eating. In view of this he thought it appropriate not to take any insulin.

Results—While the patient was receiving 85% oxygen by a non-rebreathing mask with reservoir, an arterial sample was taken for blood gas analysis. The results were:

Measure	Normal	Patient
pH	7·36–7·44	7·2
$PaCO_2$	35–45 mm Hg (4·7–6·0 kPa)	22 mm Hg (2·9 kPa)
Actual HCO_3^-	21–28 mmol/l	5·4 mmol/l
Standard HCO_3^-	21–27 mmol/l	7·5 mmol/l
Base excess	±2 mmol/l	−26 mmol/l

Analysis—Considering the history, this patient is at risk of developing a metabolic acidosis from two sources. Firstly, he could develop diabetic ketoacidosis because he is not taking his insulin and therefore unable to metabolise glucose properly. This will cause his body to metabolise fat excessively and so produce ketone bodies (the main ones are acetoacetic and β-hydroxy butyric acids), which are strongly acidic. Secondly, he may have also developed a lactic acidosis due to hypovolaemia resulting from fluid loss from sweating and polyuria.

Do the results support this clinical proposal? The answer to this is yes because:

- The pH is low, indicating there is an acidaemia
- The standard bicarbonate is low, indicating there is a metabolic acidosis
- The base excess is extremely negative, indicating the body is having to use all of its extracellular buffers to take up the extra hydrogen ions*
- The $PaCO_2$ is low indicating respiratory compensation.

Putting these all together you can conclude that this patient has developed a metabolic acidosis, and the body has compensated by increasing the respiratory rate and therefore blowing off additional carbon dioxide. In addition, over the three days we would expect the kidneys to have adapted by excreting hydrogen ions and retaining increasing amounts of bicarbonate. Nevertheless, these compensations remain only partial, and the patient is therefore still acidaemic.

Combined metabolic and respiratory acidosis

If both the metabolic and respiratory systems are defective or inadequate to the body's needs then the accumulation of acid and

* If you are unclear about the difference between base excess and standard bicarbonate, see pages 33–34.

carbon dioxide will be unchecked once the body's buffers are used up. Two common examples of this particularly dire situation are patients with cardiogenic shock and those suffering from cardiorespiratory arrest. In both cases the cells of the body produce excessive amounts of lactic acid because they are being starved of oxygen. In addition, carbon dioxide accumulates in the cells and the blood because it can no longer be removed by the lungs because of the lack of ventilation (figure 5.8).

An arterial blood sample taken at this time would therefore demonstate a combined respiratory and metabolic acidosis:

Measure	Normal	Respiratory and metabolic acidaemia
pH	7·36–7·44	↓↓↓↓
$PaCO_2$	35–45 mm Hg (4·7–6·0 kPa)	↑↑
Actual HCO_3^-	21–28 mmol/l	↓
Standard HCO_3^-	21–27 mmol/l	↓↓
Base excess	±2 mmol/l	↓↓

Figure 5.9 depicts these changes for those who like to use graphs. The graph shows clearly that patients with a combined acidosis do not fit into any of the bands drawn previously.

Halt: Key point

Combined acidosis results do not fit into the normal distribution bands for simple metabolic or respiratory acidosis

Self evidently patients who are suffering from a cardiorespiratory arrest require immediate resuscitation. Consequently, arterial samples for blood gas analysis should be taken only after adequate ventilation has been started. This has the effect of correcting the respiratory acidosis (by eliminating the excess carbon dioxide) but leaving the metabolic acidosis. To help put these changes into context, consider the following clinical examples

Example 7

History—A 68 year old man was brought to the emergency department complaining of chest pain and shortness of breath. He

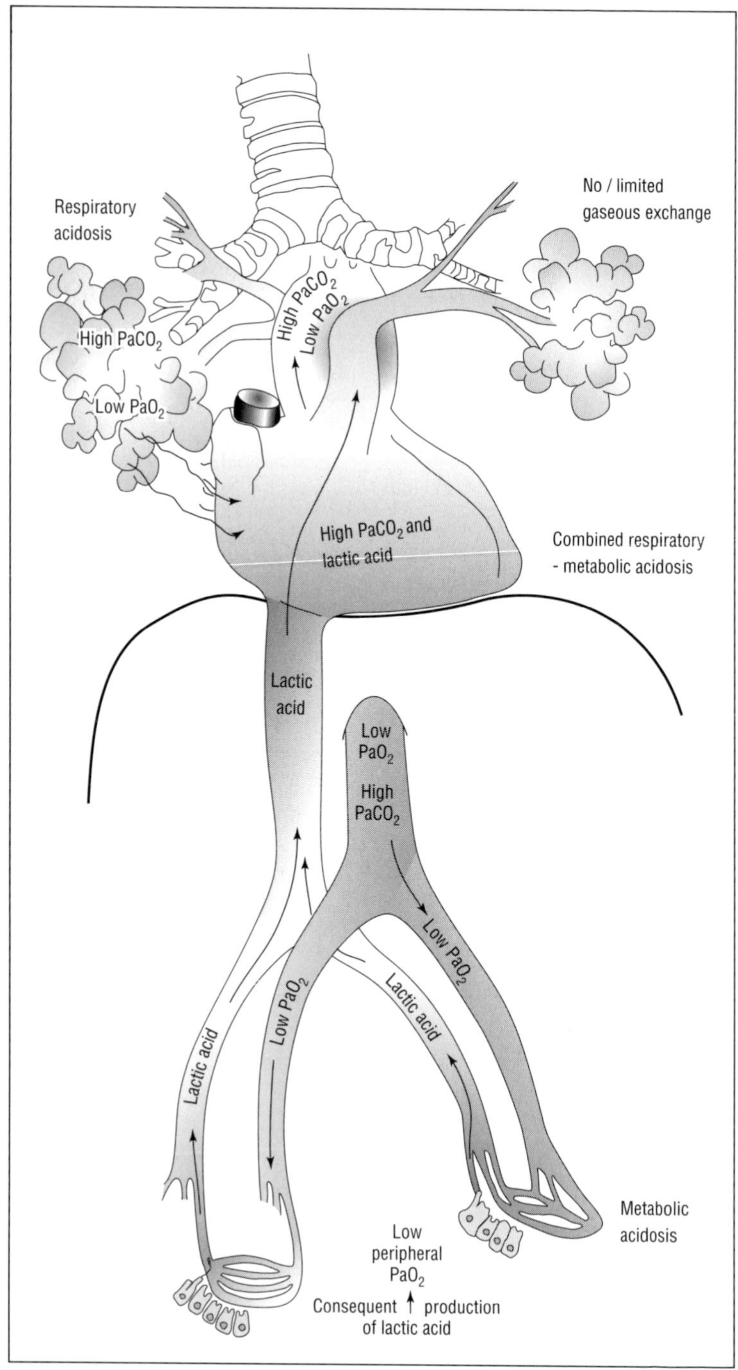

Figure 5.8 Combined respiratory and metabolic acidosis.

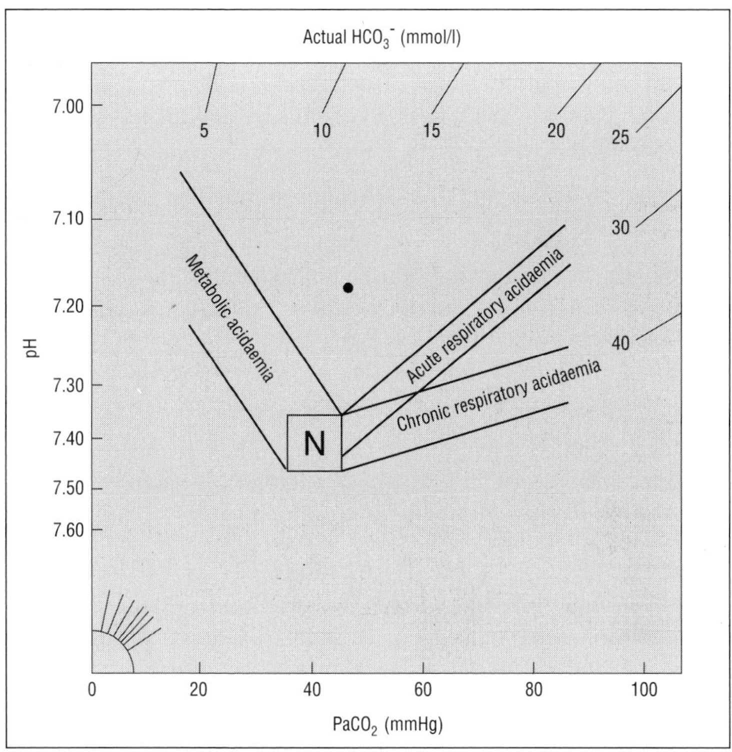

Figure 5.9 Results from a patient with a combined respiratory and metabolic acidaemia (●) superimposed on figure 5.7.

was pale, cold, and clammy, and further examination confirmed that he was in biventricular failure. His breathing was laboured with a respiratory rate of 8/min.

Results—While the patient was breathing 85% oxygen by a non-rebreathing mask with reservoir, an arterial sample was taken for blood gas analysis. The results were:

Measure	Normal	Patient
pH	7·36–7·44	6·99
$PaCO_2$	35–45 mm Hg (4·7–6·0 kPa)	109·5 mm Hg (14·6 kPa)
Actual HCO_3^-	21–28 mmol/l	15·5 mmol/l
Standard HCO_3^-	21–27 mmol/l	15·3 mmol/l
Base excess	±2 mmol/l	−12·4 mmol/l

Analysis—This patient's $PaCO_2$ was bound to be high because his ventilation was inadequate. In addition, he was showing the signs of poor peripheral perfusion (pale, cold, and clammy), indicating that his body was likely to be producing excessive amounts of lactic acid.

Do the results support this clinical proposal? The answer to this is yes because:

- The pH is low, indicating there is an acidaemia
- The $PaCO_2$ is very high, indicating there is a respiratory acidosis
- The standard bicarbonate is low and the base excess clearly negative, indicating there is a metabolic acidosis.

Putting these all together you can conclude that this man has a combined respiratory and metabolic acidosis. These have led to a large drop in the patient's pH.

Example 8

History—A 66 year old woman was admitted to the emergency department having collapsed at home. Clinical examination confirmed she was in cardiorespiratory arrest and electrocardiography showed ventricular fibrillation. Basic and advanced cardiopulmonary resuscitation was therefore started.

Results—While the patient was being ventilated with 100% oxygen, an arterial sample was taken for blood gas analysis. The results were:

Measure	Normal	Patient
pH	7·36–7·44	6·86
$PaCO_2$	35–45 mm Hg (4·7–6·0 kPa)	38·9 mm Hg (5·2 kPa)
Actual HCO_3^-	21–28 mmol/l	6·6 mmol/l
Standard HCO_3^-	21–27 mmol/l	6·6 mmol/l
Base excess	±2 mmol/l	−23·9 mmol/l

Analysis—The history indicates that this woman may have developed a combined respiratory and metabolic acidosis. If the patient is being adequately ventilated, however, then the excess carbon dioxide is likely to have been eliminated. In contrast, the metabolic acidosis will still be present because tissue perfusion will remain poor even with good cardiopulmonary resuscitation.

Do the results support this clinical proposal? The answer to this is yes because:

- The pH is low, indicating there is an acidaemia.
- The $PaCO_2$ is normal, indicating that artificial ventilation has corrected the respiratory acidosis.
- The standard bicarbonate is low and the base excess clearly negative, indicating there is a metabolic acidosis.

Putting these all together you can conclude that the artificial ventilation is sufficient to correct the respiratory acidosis. This patient retains a metabolic acidosis, however, which is big enough to cause a large change in the pH.

Summary

This chapter has concentrated on the common types of acidosis you will encounter in your clinical practice. A respiratory acidosis gives rise to an increase in the partial pressure of carbon dioxide in the extracellular fluid. Over time this is compensated for by the kidneys, which retain more bicarbonate. This therefore gives rise to an increase in standard bicarbonate concentration as well as the base excess. In the acute situation this metabolic compensation is not complete and so the pH is still below the normal range. If the respiratory acidosis is long standing, however, the compensation may be complete. In this situation the pH will be within the normal range even though the $PaCO_2$, standard bicarbonate, and base excess concentrations are higher than normal.

Metabolic acidosis causes the bicarbonate concentration to fall. The respiratory component of the body's acid base balance helps by lowering the carbon dioxide concentration as a result of increasing the respiratory rate. This, however, lowers the bicarbonate concentration further but does allow the pH to move closer to the normal range. Provided the kidneys are not the cause of the metabolic acidosis, bicarbonate will be increasingly retained over the next few days so helping to balance the acid load even further. This slightly reduces the respiratory stimulus, and so the $PaCO_2$ rises. Throughout these early and late stages it is rare for the body to overcompensate. Consequently, the pH is invariably below the normal range but rises slowly as further compensation comes into effect.

When there is a combined respiratory and metabolic acidosis the body no longer has any compensation available other than its buffers. These rapidly become saturated and therefore ineffective. Therefore the pH falls sharply, and this is accompanied by evidence of the underlying respiratory acidosis (that is, an increase in $PaCO_2$) and underlying metabolic acidosis (fall in the standard bicarbonate and base excess concentrations).

Quiz

This chapter has discussed many of the fundamental principles underlying the acidotic cases you will commonly come across. Go for a run and think about what you have read. When you come back (and have had a shower!) take the opportunity to test your comprehension by having a go at quiz 5 below.

Quiz 5 (answers on page 154–6)

1 **What happens to the $PaCO_2$ in respiratory acidosis?**
2 **What is the difference between partial and complete compensation?**
3 **What are the three main ways of producing a metabolic acidosis?**
4 **What happens to the standard bicarbonate concentration and base excess in a metabolic acidosis?**
5 **What two types of compensation are possible in metabolic acidosis?**
6 **What effect do these two types of compensation for metabolic acidosis have on the actual bicarbonate concentration?**
7 **What is the body's only remaining defence agains the acid load encountered during a cardiac arrest?**
8 **What acid-base disturbance is present in the following clinical example?**

History—A previously well 80 year old woman was brought into the emergency department after being found unconscious at home. On examination she was unresponsive and seemed to have suffered an intracerebral haemorrhage.

Results—While the patient was receiving 85% oxygen by a non-rebreathing mask with a reservoir, an arterial sample was taken for blood gas analysis. The results were:

Measure	Normal	Patient
pH	7·36–7·44	7·06
$PaCO_2$	35–45 mm Hg (4·7–6·0 kPa)	118 mm Hg (15·7 kPa)
Actual HCO_3^-	21–28 mmol/l	32·5 mmol/l
Standard HCO_3^-	21–27 mmol/l	28·4 mmol/l
Base excess	±2 mmol/l	+4 mmol/l

9 What acid-base disturbance is present in the following clinical example?

History—A 64 year old woman was referred to you by the GP because she had a persistent productive cough and a gradual increase in breathlessness. She had smoked 30–40 cigarettes a day for many years but had cut down recently because of her breathlessness.

Results—While the patient was breathing room air, an arterial sample was taken for blood gas analysis. The results were:

Measure	Normal	Patient
pH	7·36–7·44	7·38
$PaCO_2$	35–45 mm Hg (4·7–6·0 kPa)	63·2 mm Hg (8·4 kPa)
Actual HCO_3^-	21–28 mmol/l	37·0 mmol/l
Standard HCO_3^-	21–27 mmol/l	33·4 mmol/l
Base excess	±2 mmol/l	+5·3 mmol/l

10 What acid-base disturbance is present in the following clinical example?

History—You are called to the ward to see a 40 year old woman who had taken an overdose of dothiepin (a tricyclic antidepressant) two hours previously. She was unconscious and had a shallow breathing pattern with a rate of 8/min.

Results—While the patient was receiving 85% oxygen by a non-rebreathing mask with a reservoir bag, an arterial sample was taken for blood gas analysis. The results were:

Measure	Normal	Patient
pH	7·36–7·44	6·76
$PaCO_2$	35–45 mm Hg (4·7–6·0 kPa)	46·5 mm Hg (6·2 kPa)
Actual HCO_3^-	21–28 mmol/l	6·5 mmol/l
Standard HCO_3^-	21–27 mmol/l	6·2 mmol/l
Base excess	±2 mmol/l	−29·1 mmol/l

6 Common alkaloses

PETER DRISCOLL

Objectives

- To describe the mechanisms and causes of common respiratory and metabolic alkaloses
- To discuss how the body compensates for an alkalotic state
- To provide clinical examples of these two types of acid-base disturbance.

Respiratory alkalosis

Think back to chapter 3. In the lungs there is an exchange of the gases in the alveoli with those in the surrounding pulmonary blood vessels (figure 6.1). As a result oxygen moves into the circulation and carbon dioxide moves into the alveoli. If the respiratory rate increases or if the respiration becomes abnormally deep then the elimination of carbon dioxide can be greatly increased provided the alveolar membrane and circulation are relatively normal.

A consequence of the fall in carbon dioxide is a reduction in free hydrogen ions:

$$H^+\downarrow + HCO_3^-\downarrow \leftrightarrow H_2CO_3 \leftrightarrow CO_2\downarrow + H_2O$$

The fall in bicarbonate concentration is very small—that is, in the order of a few mmol/l. This is in contrast with the large change in pH that can result from a small reduction in the hydrogen ion concentration.*

As mentioned above the reduction in hydrogen ion concentration results from a fall in the concentration of carbon dioxide secondary to a defect in the respiratory system (figure 6.2). Therefore this process is called a **respiratory alkalosis**. This is much less common than respiratory acidosis and is brought about by either respiratory stimulation or loss of the normal respiratory

* If this paragraph is confusing you, reread the section on pH (page 23).

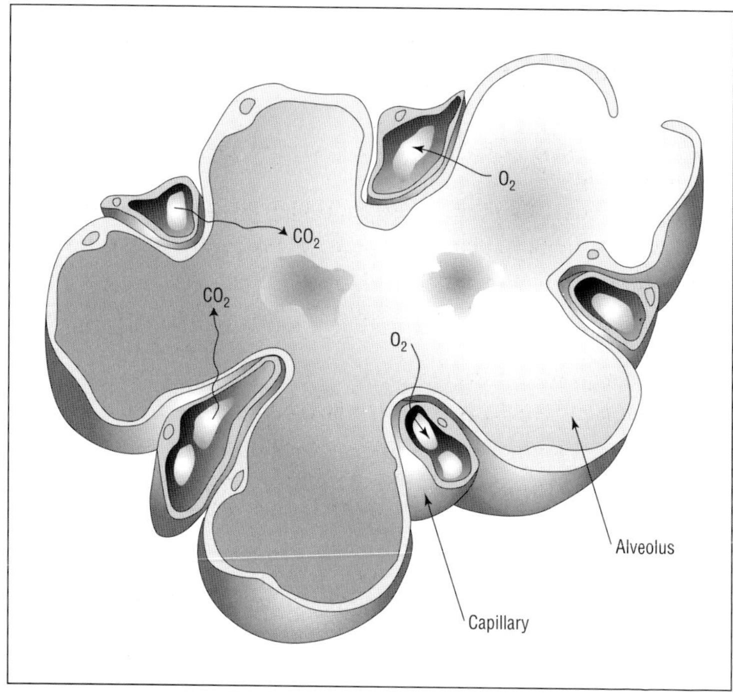

Figure 6.1 Gas exchange at alveoli.

feedback control. There are therefore many causes for it, but the end result in all cases is a fall in the $PaCO_2$ (box 6.1) (figure 6.2). If the pH rises above the normal range as a result of this then a **respiratory alkalaemia** will have been produced.

Acute respiratory alkalosis

If an arterial blood sample was taken from a patient with an acute respiratory alkalosis the following result would be obtained:

Measure	Normal	Respiratory alkalaemia
pH	7·36–7·44	↑↑
$PaCO_2$	35–45 mm Hg (4·7–6·0 kPa)	↓↓
Actual HCO_3^-	21–28 mmol/l	↓
Standard HCO_3^-	21–27 mmol/l	21–27 mmol/l
Base excess	±2 mmol/l	±2 mmol/l

As with acidosis, the body's initial response to this acid-base

Box 6.1 Common causes of hyperventilation leading to respiratory alkalosis

A fall in oxygen

- Severe anaemia, pulmonary disease, septicaemia, congestive heart failure, high altitude

The detection of a pulmonary pathology by lung receptors

- Lobar pneumonia, pulmonary oedema, pulmonary emboli

Stimulation of central nervous system

- Voluntary hyperventilation—overriding normal respiratory control
- Gram negative septicaemia
- Respiratory stimulants—for example, salicylate overdose
- Rapid correction of metabolic acidosis with bicarbonate
- Cerebral disturbance—for example, raised intracranial pressure, trauma, infection, pontine tumours, cerebrovascular haemorrhage

Miscellaneous

- Mechanical hyperventilation—for example, overenthusiastic manual ventilation or setting the ventilator so that it delivers an excessively high respiratory rate

disturbance is to use its buffers. Within 10 minutes intracellular and extracellular proteins release hydrogen ions into the extracellular fluid to try to normalise the pH. In addition, the kidneys will help by increasing the excretion of bicarbonate in the urine and retaining hydrogen ions. This takes 2–5 days to reach an optimal level and is known as metabolic compensation.

If an arterial blood sample was taken once the metabolic compensation had occurred, the following result would be obtained:

Measure	Normal	Respiratory alkalaemia	Metabolic compensation
pH	7·36–7·44	↑↑	↑
$PaCO_2$	35–45 mm Hg (4·7–6·0 kPa)	↓↓	↓↓
Actual HCO_3^-	21–28 mmol/l	↓	↓↓
Standard HCO_3^-	21–27 mmol/l	21·27 mmol/l	↓
Base excess	±2 mmol/l	±2 mmol/l	↓

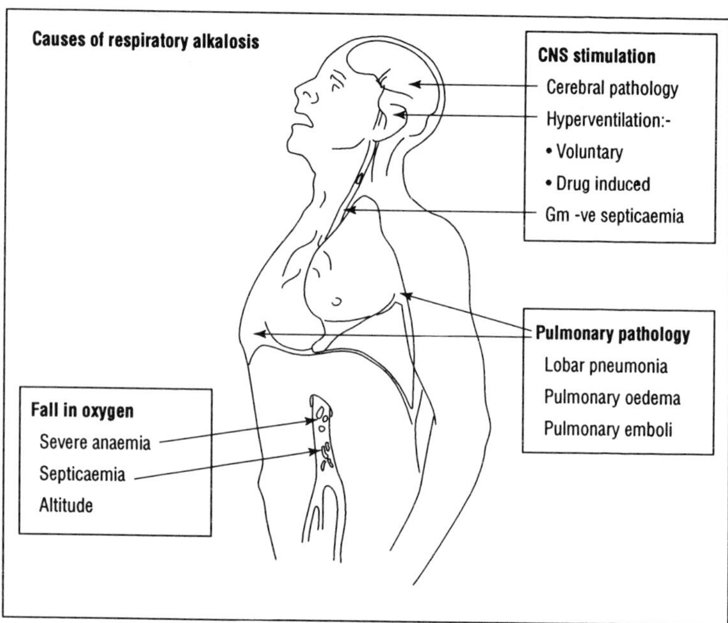

Figure 6.2 Causes of respiratory alkalosis.

Usually respiratory alkaloses do not last long enough for full metabolic compensation to develop. Consequently, the pH is still high but it is closer to the normal range.

These changes can be demonstrated in graphical form (figure 6.3).

Halt: Key points

- **Respiratory alkalosis is associated with a fall in $PaCO_2$**
- **The metabolic component of the body's acid-base balance can compensate for a respiratory alkalosis by increasing the loss of bicarbonate**
- **Metabolic compensation usually takes 2–5 days to achieve an optimal level**

To put these changes into context it is helpful to review a clinical case.

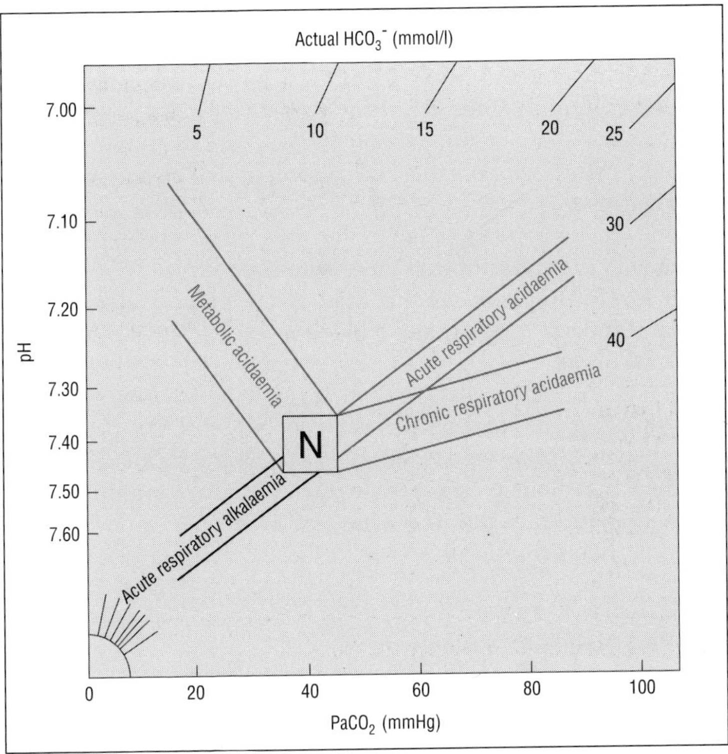

Figure 6.3 The possible ranges associated with acute respiratory alkalaemia superimposed on figure 5.7.

Example 1

History—A 16 year old girl was admitted to hospital after an argument with her boyfriend. She denied taking any medication. On examination her chest was clear but her respiratory rate was 34/minute.

Results—While she was breathing room air, an arterial sample was taken for blood gas analysis. The results were:

Measure	Normal	Patient
pH	7·36–7·44	7·5
$PaCO_2$	35–45 mm Hg (4·7–6·0 kPa)	27 mm Hg (3·6 kPa)
Actual HCO_3^-	21–28 mmol/l	20·5 mmol/l
Standard HCO_3^-	21–27 mmol/l	23·1 mmol/l
Base excess	±2 mmol/l	– 1·0 mmol/l

Analysis—A normal respiratory rate in a girl of this age would be around 12–18/min at rest. Therefore from what you have read so far in this chapter you would expect this girl to have a respiratory alkalosis as a result of the greatly increased respiratory rate.

Do the results support this clinical proposal? The answer to this is yes because:

- The high pH confirms that there is an alkalaemia
- The low $PaCO_2$ indicates that there is a respiratory alkalosis
- The standard bicarbonate and base excess are both within normal limits.

Putting these all together you can conclude that this patient has developed an alkalaemia secondary to a respiratory alkalosis. As the standard bicarbonate and base excess levels are within normal limits, this indicates that there has not been time to develop any metabolic compensation.

Chronic respiratory alkalosis

If the cause of the respiratory alkalosis lasts over three days metabolic compensation will be detected. In these cases the patient's pH is moved closer to the normal range. Indeed if the body is able to develop full compensation the pH will be within the normal range. As with chronic respiratory acidosis, however, this does not mean that the $PaCO_2$ and HCO_3^- concentration will be normal.

The following clinical example also helps to demonstrate these changes.

Example 2

History—A 52 year old man was brought into the emergency department complaining of a cough and pleuritic chest pain for several days. He had also noticed that he was increasingly short of breath.

Results—While the patient was breathing 30% oxygen by mask, an arterial sample was taken for blood gas analysis. The results were:

Measure	Normal	Patient
pH	7·36–7·44	7·52
$PaCO_2$	35–45 mm Hg (4·7–6·0 kPa)	13·7 mm Hg (1·8 kPa)
Actual HCO_3^-	21–28 mmol/l	12·2 mmol/l
Standard HCO_3^-	21–27 mmol/l	14·1 mmol/l
Base excess	±2 mmol/l	−8·2 mmol/l

Analysis—A history of feeling short of breath for the past few days, combined with pleuritic chest pain, will tend to cause the patient to breathe rapidly and shallowly. As a result we would expect him to lower his $PaCO_2$. As this had been going on for some days we would also expect to see evidence of metabolic compensation.

Do the results support this clinical proposal? The answer to this is yes because:

- The high pH confirms there is an alkalaemia
- The low $PaCO_2$ indicates that there is a respiratory alkalosis
- Both the standard bicarbonate and base excess are lowered.

Putting these all together you can conclude that this patient has developed a respiratory alkalosis. As there is no cause for a metabolic acidosis, the low standard bicarbonate and base excess concentrations indicate that the respiratory alkalosis has been going on long enough for considerable metabolic compensation to develop. Even so, the pH is still above the normal range, indicating that the compensation is only partial.

Metabolic alkalosis

This occurs when the body either loses acid or, less commonly, gains base (box 6.2).

The effect of vomiting or gastric aspiration will depend on whether there is a net loss of acid or of alkali. If it is mainly gastric contents then there is net loss of hydrogen ions, which is equivalent to giving the body a bolus of strong alkali. Intestinal contents distal to the second part of the duodenum, however, have a high concentration of bicarbonate. Consequently, loss of this fluid leads to a loss of bicarbonate and a metabolic acidosis (see page 76).

A low concentration of extracellular potassium (hypokalaemia) can be dangerous because it can lead to a life threatening failure of muscle contractility. The body can compensate by releasing

Box 6.2 Causes of metabolic alkalosis

Losing acid

- Gastrointestinal loss—for example, vomiting (prolonged vomiting is the commonest cause of metabolic alkalosis), gastric aspiration
- Hydrogen movement into cells—for example, hypokalaemia
- Renal loss—for example, after diuretic treatment

Gaining base

- Iatrogenic—for example, inappropriate treatment of acidosis
- Chronic alkali ingestion – for example, the milk alkali syndrome

potassium ions from cells but only if hydrogen ions move in the opposite direction—that is, into the cells of the body (figure 6.4). As a result, this exchange causes intracellular acidosis and extracellular alkalosis.

A fall in plasma concentration can occur for a variety of reasons. A particularly common one is an increased loss of potassium in the urine after loop or thiazide diuretic treatment. This movement of potassium is accompanied by an increased uptake in bicarbonate by the renal tubules. As a result the patient's bicarbonate concentration increases and a metabolic alkalosis can develop.

There are additional ways in which these types of diuretics can produce a metabolic alkalosis. Firstly, they increase the rate of flow through the renal tubules and as a result increase the loss of hydrogen ions into the urine. Secondly, they also cause a fall in the extracellular fluid, sodium, and chloride. The body adapts to these changes by increasing its production of the hormone aldosterone. This helps to preserve the blood volume by increasing the reabsorption of sodium from the lumen of the renal tubules. Like the situation with potassium above, however, the movement of sodium is linked with the loss of hydrogen ions into the lumen of the renal tubule (figure 6.5). Bicarbonate is produced along with the hydrogen ions. When these hydrogen ions are lost into the lumen, bicarbonate moves into the blood stream.

Halt: Key point

The more sodium that is reabsorbed the more alkalotic the patient will become

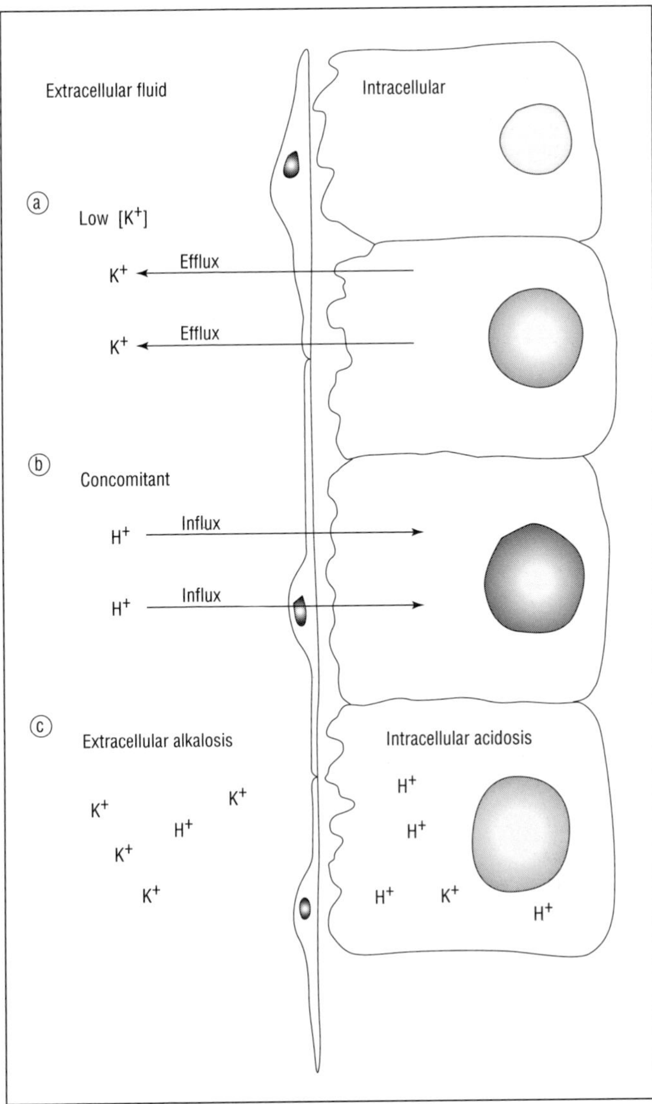

Figure 6.4 Exchange of hydrogen ions for potassium by cells, resulting in an extracellular alkalosis.

The end result from all the causes of metabolic alkalosis is that the blood's bicarbonate concentration rises whereas its hydrogen ion concentration falls. As these changes are due to a defect in the metabolic component of the body's acid-base balance, this process is called a **metabolic alkalosis**. The term **metabolic alkalaemia** would be used if this fall in the hydrogen ion concentration was sufficient to cause the pH to rise above the normal range.

Acute metabolic alkalosis

If an arterial sample was taken when a metabolic alkalosis had just started then the following result would be obtained:

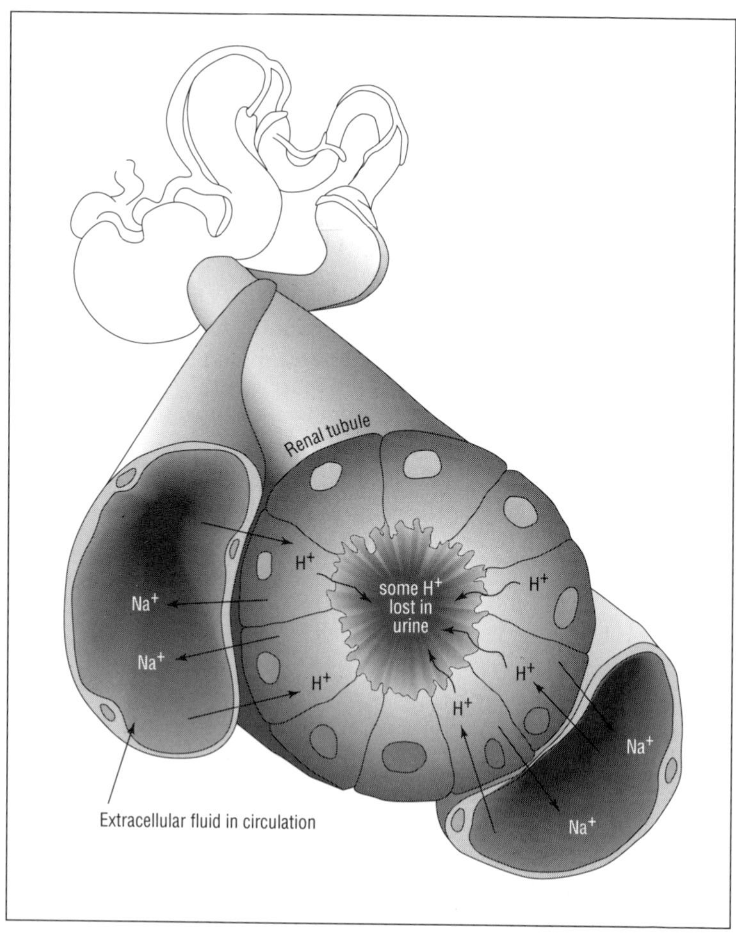

Figure 6.5 Sodium/hydrogen ion link in renal tubular cells with the loss of hydrogen ions into urine.

Measure	Normal	Metabolic alkalaemia
pH	7·36–7·44	↑↑
$PaCO_2$	35–45 mm Hg (4·7–6·0 kPa)	35–45 mm Hg (4·7–6·0 kPa)
Actual HCO_3^-	21–28 mmol/l	↑↑
Standard HCO_3^-	21–27 mmol/l	↑↑
Base excess	±2 mmol/l	↑↑

As with respiratory alkalosis, buffers will be used to try to correct the fall in hydrogen ion concentration. In addition, by means of the respiratory-metabolic link the lungs can help by reducing the respiratory rate and retaining carbon dioxide. This respiratory compensation begins within minutes and is complete within 12–24 hours. It has the effect of increasing the production of hydrogen ions from the breakdown of carbonic acid:

$$\xleftarrow{\hspace{6cm}}$$
$$H^+\uparrow + HCO_3^-\uparrow \leftrightarrow H_2CO_3 \leftrightarrow CO_2\uparrow + H_2O$$

As bicarbonate is also generated by this reaction there is a small rise in the actual bicarbonate concentration. The following results would therefore be obtained if an arterial blood sample was taken once the respiratory compensation had occurred:

Measure	Normal	Metabolic alkalaemia	Respiratory compensation
pH	7·36–7·44	↑↑	↑
$PaCO_2$	35–45 mm Hg (4·7–6·0 kPa)	35–45 mm Hg (4·7–6·0 kPa)	↑↑↑
Actual HCO_3^-	21–28 mmol/l	↑↑	↑↑↑
Standard HCO_3^-	21–27 mmol/l	↑↑	↑↑
Base excess	±2 mmol/l	↑↑	↑↑

The body will limit the degree of respiratory compensation possibly because this depends on reducing ventilation and thereby lowering the arterial partial pressure of oxygen. In alkalaemic patients, however, the PaO_2 would have to fall to below 50–60 mm Hg (6·7–8·0 kPa) before ventilation is stimulated and further respiratory compensation curtailed. This means that respiratory compensation can cause the $PaCO_2$ to rise to as much as 60 mm Hg (8·0 kPa) in previously normal patients with severe metabolic alkalosis.

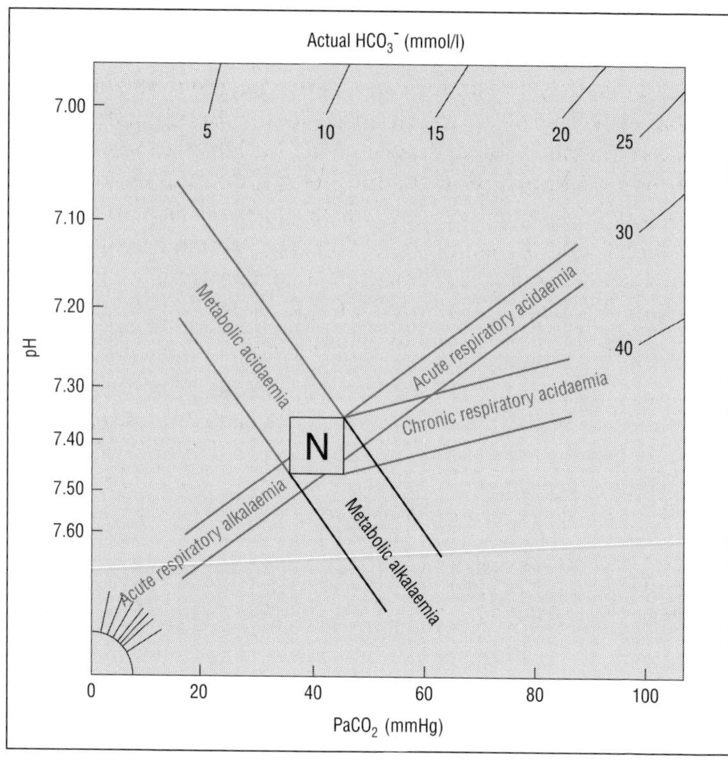

Figure 6.6 The possible ranges associated with metabolic alkalaemia superimposed on figure 6.3.

These changes are depicted on figure 6.6.

Halt: Key points

- **Metabolic alkalosis is associated with a rise in the concentrations of both the standard bicarbonate and base excess**
- **The respiratory component of the body's acid-base balance can compensate for a metabolic alkalosis by retaining carbon dioxide**
- **Respiratory compensation usually starts within minutes and takes 12–24 hours to achieve a maximal level**

Chronic metabolic alkalosis

If the metabolic alkalosis persists the kidneys will adapt, provided that they are not the cause of the metabolic alkalosis. This adaptation will result in an increased loss of bicarbonate and an increased retention of hydrogen ions. In other words there is **metabolic compensation for the metabolic alkalosis**. As with previous renal adaptations this will take several days to develop. During this time the stimulus to alter the respiratory pattern will decrease, allowing the respiratory rate to increase and the $PaCO_2$ to fall slighly. Therefore, if an arterial blood sample was taken at this stage the following result would be obtained:

Measure	Normal	Metabolic alkalaemia	Respiratory compensation	Metabolic compensation
pH	7·36–7·44	↑↑	↑	↑
$PaCO_2$	35–45 mm Hg (4·7–6·0 kPa)	35–45 mm Hg (4·7–6·0 kPa)	↑↑↑	↑↑
Actual HCO_3^-	21–28 mmol/l	↑↑	↑↑↑	↑↑
Standard HCO_3^-	21–27 mmol/l	↑↑	↑↑	↑
Base excess	±2 mmol/l	↑↑	↑↑	↑

It is important to be aware that the degree of renal compensation may be limited by the demand to retain electrolytes and fluid. For example, if the metabolic alkalosis was due to persistent vomiting then there would also be associated fluid and electrolyte loss. In this situation the retention of sodium would take priority over acid-base homeostasis. As a result the kidney will excrete hydrogen and potassium ions and retain sodium, chloride, and bicarbonate. The loss of hydrogen and potassium ions in the urine along with the retention of bicarbonate will obviously make the metabolic alkalosis worse.

To help demonstrate these points consider the following example.

Example 3

History—A 26 year old man presented to the emergency department with a four day history of vomiting after his return from a holiday abroad. He had slight diarrhoea.

Results—While the patient was breathing room air, an arterial sample was taken for blood gas analysis. The results were:

Measure	Normal	Patient
pH	7·36–7·44	7·48
$PaCO_2$	35–45 mm Hg (4·7–6·0 kPa)	43·6 mm Hg (5·8 kPa)
Actual HCO_3^-	21–28 mmol/l	31·5 mmol/l
Standard HCO_3^-	21–27 mmol/l	30 mmol/l
Base excess	±2 mmol/l	+4·5 mmol/l

Analysis—As described above, persistent vomiting of gastric contents leads to the loss of hydrochloric acid from the stomach. As a result, there are fewer free hydrogen ions in the circulation and an alkalaemia develops. The body tries to compensate by retaining carbon dioxide. If the patient does not have an electrolyte imbalance the body will also increase the excretion of bicarbonate from the kidneys and retain hydrogen ions.

This patient has been vomiting for several days. Consequently his acid-base status will depend on which factors predominate—that is, the loss of acid, the loss of fluid, or electrolyte abnormalities. In this case, we can see that the main problem has been the loss of acid because:

- The pH is high, indicating an alkalaemia
- The $PaCO_2$ is at the upper end of normal, indicating an early move toward respiratory compensation
- Both the standard bicarbonate and base excess are raised, indicating there is a metabolic alkalosis.

Initially the management of any type of metabolic alkalosis is directed at treating the underlying cause. If the vomiting persists, however, hypovolaemia could occur along with the considerable loss of essential electrolytes. In this situation the body will change its priorities such that retaining essential electrolytes will take preference over maintaining the acid-base balance.

It follows therefore that if your are managing a patient who is in this clinical state then you must aim to correct the deficiencies in the essential electrolytes first. Consequently, you need to start by giving an infusion of isotonic sodium chloride. In so doing you replace the extracellular fluid loss and restore the sodium and chloride concentations. This enables the body to switch from dealing with retaining essential electrolytes to correcting the underlying alkalosis. In other words, by giving the patient essential electrolytes you allow the body to put its own "acid-base" house in order.

Example 4

History—An 81 year old woman who was known to have ischaemic heart disease developed ankle oedema. She was subsequently treated with bendrofluazide (a thiazide diuretic) prescribed by her general practitioner. After a further attack of angina she presented to the emergency department.

Results—While the patient was breathing room air, an arterial sample was taken for blood gas analysis. The results were:

Measure	Normal	Patient
pH	7·36–7·44	7·54
$PaCO_2$	35–45 mm Hg (4·7–6·0 kPa)	50·2 mm Hg (6·7 kPa)
Actual HCO_3^-	21–28 mmol/l	44·0 mmol/l
Standard HCO_3^-	21–27 mmol/l	37·0 mmol/l
Base excess	±2 mmol/l	+17 mmol/l

Analysis—For the reasons described previously, diuretics such as bendrofluazide can lead to metabolic alkalosis. If this had occurred, however, we would expect the patient to demonstrate evidence of respiratory compensation.

Do the results support our clinical suspicions? The answer is yes because:

- The pH is high, indicating an alkalaemia
- The high $PaCO_2$ is in keeping with respiratory compensation
- The standard bicarbonate and base excess are raised, indicating there is a metabolic alkalosis.

Summary

Respiratory alkalosis leads to a fall in the $PaCO_2$. It can be caused by several conditions, but it is usually short lived. In those cases when it does persist the body will mount a metabolic compensatory response in which the kidneys will retain hydrogen ions from the urine and increase the removal of bicarbonate.

In contrast, metabolic alkaloses cause the bicarbonate concentration to rise either because of a loss of acid or because more base has been taken into the body. The body will respond quickly by utilising the respiratory component of the acid-base balance. This results in a reduction in alveolar ventilation so that carbon dioxide is retained. Later provided the kidneys are functioning properly, a metabolic compensatory response will also develop. This will help to remove some of the excess bicarbonate and retain extra hydrogen ions. It is important to be aware, however, that both the initial respiratory compensation and the later metabolic compensation can be limited by other factors. Consequently, the pH may be only partially restored.

Quiz

This chapter has discussed many of the fundamental principles underlying the alkalotic cases you will commonly come across. Go and make another coffee and think for a few minutes about what you have read. When you come back take the opportunity to test your comprehension by having a go at quiz 6 below.

Quiz 6 (answers on pages 156–7)

1. **What happens to the $PaCO_2$ in patients with respiratory alkalosis?**
2. **What is the difference between respiratory alkalosis and respiratory alkalaemia?**
3. **It is normal to have well developed metabolic compensation to a respiratory alkalosis?**
4. **Which is the commonest cause of metabolic alkalosis—loss of acid or base gain?**
5. **What happens to the actual bicarbonate concentration after respiratory compensation to a metabolic alkalosis?**
6. **What is the factor limiting the respiratory response to metabolic alkalosis?**
7. **What factors can limit the metabolic response to metabolic alkalosis?**
8. **What acid-base disturbance is present in the following clinical example?**

History—A 51 year old woman presented to the emergency department complaining of shortness of breath. This symptom had been going on for years, and she wanted it to stop. She had no other medical problems. On examination she had a resting respiratory rate of 20/min.

Results—While the patient was breathing room air, an arterial sample was taken for blood gas analysis. The results were:

Measure	Normal	Patient
pH	7·36–7·44	7·48
$PaCO_2$	35–45 mm Hg (4·7–6·0 kPa)	17·9 mm Hg (2·4 kPa)
Actual HCO_3^-	21–28 mmol/l	12·5 mmol/l
Standard HCO_3^-	21–27 mmol/l	14·5 mmol/l
Base excess	±2 mmol/l	− 6·6 mmol/l

9 What acid-base disturbance is present in the following clinical example?

History—For 10 days after a cholecystectomy, a 69 year old woman had had a paralytic ileus. During this time she had been having regular gastric aspiration from a nasogastric tube.

Results—While the patient was breathing room air, an arterial sample was taken for blood gas analysis. The results were:

Measure	Normal	Patient
pH	7·36–7·44	7·58
$PaCO_2$	35–45 mm Hg (4·7–6·0 kPa)	53·1 mm Hg (7·1 kPa)
Actual HCO_3^-	21–28 mmol/l	49·0 mmol/l
Standard HCO_3^-	21–27 mmol/l	46·0 mmol/l
Base excess	2 mmol/l	+20 mmol/l

10 What acid-base disturbance is present in the following clinical example?

History—A 43 year old publican had a history of alcoholic liver disease. He had recently developed ascites that failed to respond to oral bumetanide (a loop diuretic).

Results—While the patient was receiving 28% oxygen by a mask, an arterial sample was taken for blood gas analysis. The results were:

Measure	Normal	Patient
pH	7·36–7·44	7·59
$PaCO_2$	35–45 mm Hg (4·7–6·0 kPa)	61·0 mm Hg (8·1 kPa)
Actual HCO_3^-	21–28 mmol/l	56·5 mmol/l
Standard HCO_3^-	21–27 mmol/l	49·2 mmol/l
Base excess	±2 mmol/l	+25 mmol/l

7 Interpreting a blood gas sample

PETER DRISCOLL, TERRY BROWN

Objectives

- To show how the patient's overall acid-base status is determined
- To emphasise the importance of the patient's clinical history and examination
- To describe how it is possible to distinguish between single and mixed acid-base disturbances.

Take a moment to consider how you interpret the results of any clinical investigation. Commonly there are three elements (box 7.1). Firstly, you assess the patient. Secondly, you use some type of system to analyse all the information in the results. Finally, you put these two together to arrive at a conclusion. If the clinical findings and the results agree then you are usually well on the way to achieving a specific diagnosis. When they do not agree, however, the diagnosis remains unknown and further investigations and considerations will be necessary.

Interpretation of a blood gas result also includes these three elements. In fact appropriate conclusions can be drawn only by integrating the patient's clinical state with a systematic analysis of the results.

Box 7.1 Interpreting results

- Consider the patient's clinical history and physical examination
- Systematically analyse the results
- Integrate the clinical findings with the interpretation of the data

Clinical assessment

In the previous chapters the following acid-base disturbances have been discussed:

- Acute respiratory acidosis
- Chronic respiratory acidosis
- Acute metabolic acidosis
- Chronic metabolic acidosis
- Combined metabolic and respiratory acidosis
- Acute respiratory alkalosis
- Chronic respiratory alkalosis
- Acute metabolic alkalosis
- Chronic metabolic alkalosis.

Unfortunately patients do not present with a sign saying which particular acid-base disturbance they are suffering from. Instead you will have to search through all their signs and symptoms looking for clues of an underlying acid-base disturbance (box 7.2) (figure 7.1).

Box 7.2 Patient's symptoms

- Symptoms due to the cause of the acid-base disturbance
- Symptoms as a result of the acid-base disturbance
- Symptoms that have nothing to do with an acid-base disturbance

Signs and symptoms due to the cause of the acid-base disturbance

When each of the particular acid-base disturbances were discussed in previous chapters we described certain conditions that may have been the cause of the problem. To test your memory, have a go at listing the possible acid-base disturbances which may be associated with the 10 common conditions overleaf (the answers are on page 114).

- Vomiting
- Diuretic therapy
- Rapid breathing
- Diabetic coma
- Cardiac arrest
- Overdose
- Chronic antacid ingestion
- Opiate overdose
- Severe blood loss
- Chronic bronchitis.

RESPIRATORY
ACIDOSIS
Dear Dr Watson,
Thankyou for asking
me to see this man
with ? respiratory
acidosis.
Δ On review, NOT SO
elementary ...
Advise following ...

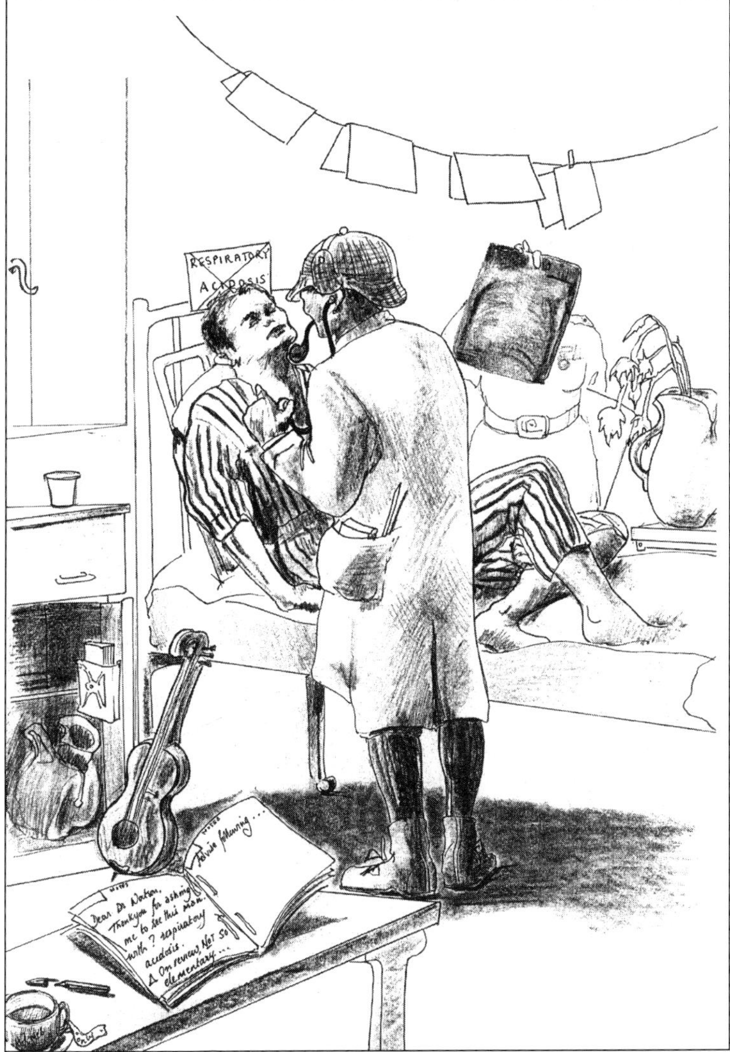

Figure 7.1 Looking for clues of an underlying acid-base disturbance.

Answers

Condition	Possible acid-base disturbances
Vomiting	Metabolic alkalosis due to loss of gastric acid Metabolic acidosis if the patient becomes hypovolaemic or if the obstruction is distal to the second part of the duodenum (see page 99)
Diuretic therapy	Metabolic alkalosis due to increased loss of hydrogen and potassium ions from the kidneys (see page 100)
Rapid breathing	Respiratory alkalosis (see page 93)
Diabetic coma	Metabolic acidosis (see page 76)
Cardiac arrest	Combined respiratory and metabolic acidosis (see page 84)
Overdose	Depends on the nature of the toxic agent but most give rise to a metabolic acidosis There could also be respiratory acidosis secondary to sedation (see page 67) or a respiratory alkalosis following salicylate overdose (see page 95)
Chronic antacid ingestion	Metabolic alkalosis (see page 100)
Opiate overdose	Acute respiratory acidosis (see page 67)
Severe blood loss	Metabolic acidosis Respiratory alkalosis secondary to hypoxia (see page 96)
Chronic bronchitis	Chronic respiratory acidosis (see page 73)

After you have checked your answers you will see that it follows therefore that if a patient presents with these conditions then you should think of the appropriate acid-base disturbance. This is particularly important when a patient has several conditions that could be having conflicting effects on the patient's overall pH. Simply analysing the results in these patients can often lead to a mixed acid-base disturbance being missed.

Signs and symptoms as a result of the acid-base disturbance

The next piece of evidence you look for to support your suspicions of an acid-base disturbance is the presence of signs and symptoms that are produced by alterations in the concentration of hydrogen ions and carbon dioxide. Let us now consider some of these.

Respiratory acidosis

Carbon dioxide retention leads to a group of symptoms of the central nervous system collectively known as "hypercapnoeic encephalopathy" (box 7.3) (figure 7.2). Overall they tend to be associated with depression of the nervous system, especially if the pH falls below 7·0.

Box 7.3 Hypercapnoeic encephalopathy

- Headache
- Irritable behaviour, progressing through to aggression
- Lack of concentration, and apathy progressing through to coma
- Confusion and incoherence through to delirium, hallucinations, and transient psychosis
- Occasionally there may be papilloedema, seizures, myoclonic jerks, flapping tremor

With mild to moderate increases of carbon dioxide various mechanisms are activated that lead to cardiovascular effects. These result in an increased cardiac output, warm skin, arrhythmias (especially supraventricular tachycardias), a bounding pulse, and sweating. If the condition persists, renal function can also be affected with the result that extra salt and water is retained. In

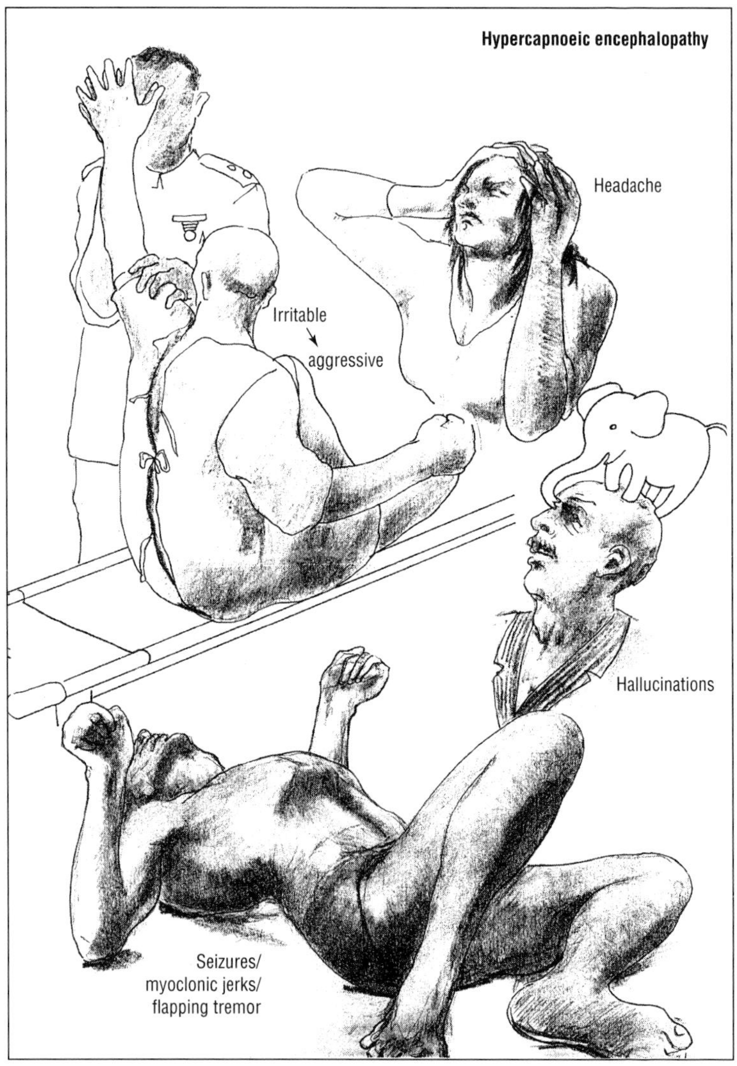

Figure 7.2 Signs of hypercapnoeic encephalopathy.

severe cases of hypercapnoea there tends to be a fall in cardiac output and hypotension.

Chronic respiratory acidosis

If the body has had time to compensate fully for the rise in $PaCO_2$ then no specific signs and symptoms will be present. If there is failure in compensation or a sudden rise in $PaCO_2$,

Box 7.4 Symptoms and signs of metabolic acidosis

- Hyperventilation ("air hunger")
- Cold, clammy skin
- Capillary stasis
- Tachycardia and arrhythmia
- Right heart strain
- Altered level of consciousness

however, then the signs and symptoms mentioned for acute respiratory acidosis will become evident.

Metabolic acidosis

We have already described that a rise in hydrogen ion concentration will lead to increased ventilation. As the minute ventilation can increase by 4–8 times, the patient may present complaining of dyspnoea. In addition to this compensatory response, there are also several other signs and symptoms resulting directly from the acidosis (box 7.4).

When there is only a mild increase in hydrogen ion concentration there is an increase in the secretion of catecholamines. As a result the strength of muscular contraction is enhanced but so is neuromuscular irritability. The latter increases the risk of arrhythmia, especially if the pH falls below 7·1. The elevated catecholamine concentration also produces a tachycardia and pale and clammy skin because of its effect on the peripheral circulation.

In cases of more severe metabolic acidosis all muscular function (including cardiac) is impaired and the blood pressure falls. There is also capillary stasis because of simultaneous arterial vasodilation and venous constriction. In addition, pulmonary vasoconstriction can occur, giving rise to right heart strain. Depression of consciousness is also found with severe acidosis, and this can lead to coma.

The rise in the concentration of hydrogen ions is often associated with an increase in the plasma concentration of potassium ions. This adds to the neuromuscular irritability and the chance of arrhythmias, such as heart block and cardiac arrest. Hyperkalaemia can also produce peaking of the T wave and broadening of the QRS complex on the electrocardiogram.

Respiratory alkalosis

This gives rise to both neurological and cardiovascular symptoms. As with a respiratory acidosis, there can be a whole collection of neurological signs. These are generally excitatory in nature and include paraesthesia (especially finger tips and lips), confusion, light headedness, and chest tightness. Rarely, there can be tetany and seizures.

The manifestations of cardiovascular symptoms depend on whether the patient is conscious or not. In the awake patient there is no appreciable effect on the cardiac output and blood pressure. In contrast, arrhythmia as well as considerable falls in the blood pressure and cardiac output can occur when acute respiratory alkalosis results from mechanical hyperventilation of patients with depressed consciousness. These changes are accompanied by increased peripheral resistance, which can give rise to high concentrations of lactic acid because of the fall in tissue perfusion (see page 76). Another cause of the fall in cardiac output in these patients is the decreased venous return resulting from the increased intrathoracic pressure.

Metabolic alkalosis

Though there are many possible signs and symptoms in a metabolic alkalosis none are specific (box 7.5). Consequently, diagnosis depends largely on clinical suspicion supported by laboratory data.

The signs of hypovolaemia (that is, reduced skin turgor, thirst, postural hypotension, decreased urine output) are usually a result of the factors giving rise to the acid-base abnormality in the first place. Nevertheless, alkalosis can also affect vascular tone, partly because of the inhibition of sympathetic discharge. In addition, the tone can also be altered by the lowering of the plasma concentra-

Box 7.5 Signs and symptoms of metabolic alkalosis

- Hypovolaemia
- Hypoventilation
- Reduction in muscle contractility
- Arrhythmia
- Altered consciousness
- Physical weakness

tion of potassium and ionised calcium, which occurs as a result of the alkalosis. In extreme cases this can lead to confusion and coma because of the effect on the cerebral circulation. It can also result in impaired coronary perfusion.

The alteration in the plasma concentrations of ionised calcium and potassium can also give rise to other effects. For example, ionised calcium is very important in neuromuscular conduction. A reduction can therefore give rise to neuromuscular irritability, tetany, muscle cramps, paraesthesia (especially finger tips and lips), impaired cardiac function, and arrhythmia. Similarly, a fall in potassium concentration reduces the contractility of all muscles. Consequently, this can give rise to ileus (smooth muscle), fatigue (skeletal muscle), and, when very low, cardiac failure (myocardium). Hypokalaemia is also associated with arrhythmia (especially tachyarrhythmias) and flattening of the T wave on electrocardiography.

Halt: Key points

Though acidosis and alkalosis can produce both coma and convulsions, in general

- **The chances of coma are higher in acidosis**
- **The chances of convulsion are higher in alkalosis**

Systematic analysis of the blood gas results

It is useful here to take a moment to remind ourselves what happens to the pH, $PaCO_2$, standard bicarbonate, and base excess in the acid-base disturbances we have discused above (table 7.1).

Looking at table 7.1 it is clear that the compensatory response is in the same direction as the primary disturbance. For example, a respiratory acidosis is caused by an increase in $PaCO_2$. The body compensates for this by increasing the concentration of bicarbonate.

Halt: Key point

The compensatory response always changes in the same direction as the primary disturbance

Table 7.1 Changes in pH, $PaCO_2$, standard bicarbonate, and base excess with common acid-base disorders*

Acid-base disorder	pH	Primary disturbance	Compensatory response
Respiratory acidosis (page 65)	↓	↑ $PaCO_2$	↑ HCO_3^- ↑ (that is, positive) base excess
Respiratory alkalosis (page 93)	↑	↓ $PaCO_2$	↓ HCO_3^- ↓ (that is, negative) base excess
Metabolic acidosis (page 76)	↓	↓ HCO_3^- ↓ (that is, negative) base excess	↓ $PaCO_2$
Metabolic alkalosis (page 101)	↑	↑ HCO_3^- ↑ (that is, positive) base excess	↑ $PaCO_2$

With this important principle in mind, we can now consider how a blood gas sample should be analysed. There are several ways for doing this in the emergency situation.

The one described below is an effective system based on a series of questions (box 7.6).

Box 7.6 Questions used in the interpretation of a blood gas sample

- Is there an acidaemia or alkalaemia?
- Is there evidence of a disturbance in the respiratory component of the body's acid-base balance?
- Is there evidence of a disturbance in the metabolic component of the body's acid-base balance?
- Is there a single or multiple acid-base disturbance?
- Is there any defect in oxygen uptake?

Is there an acidaemia or alkalaemia?

In most cases you will come across, the patient will have an acute single acid-base disturbance. In these circumstances the body has rarely had the opportunity to compensate completely for the alteration in hydrogen ion concentration. Consequently, the pH will remain outside the normal range and thereby indicate the

* If any of these come as a shock, check page 66 for respiratory acidosis, 93 for respiratory alkalosis, 76 for metabolic acidosis and 99 for metabolic alkalosis.

underlying acid-base disturbance (box 7.7)

Box 7.7 pH and the underlying acid-base disturbance

- pH less than 7·36 = underlying acidaemia
- pH greater than 7·44 = underlying alkalaemia

Halt: Key point

In acute, single acid-base disturbances the body usually does not have time to fully compensate; the pH will therefore indicate the primary acid-base problem

Nevertheless, a normal pH does not necessarily exclude an acid-base disturbance. In fact there are three reasons for a patient having a pH within the normal range:

- There is no underlying acid-base disturbance
- The body has fully compensated for a single acid-base disturbance (figure 7.3)
- There is more than one acid-base disturbance with an equal but

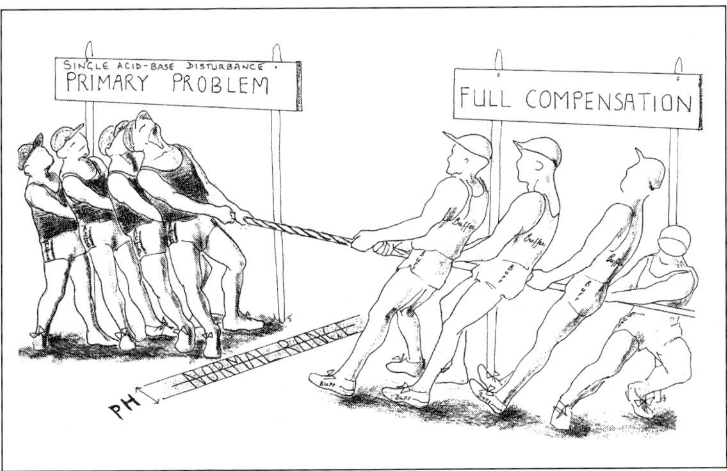

Figure 7.3 Primary problem *v* full compensation.

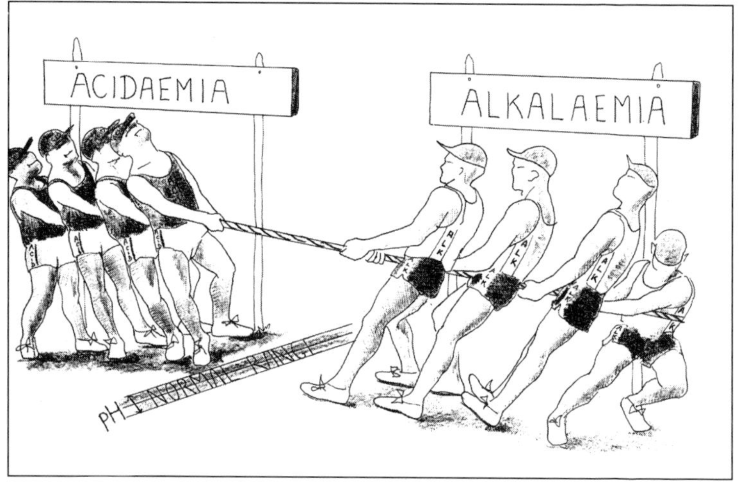

Figure 7.4 Acidaemia *v* alkalaemia.

opposite effect on the pH (figure 7.4).

By using your knowledge of the patent's clinical history and examination you will have a good idea as to which of these options is the true answer. To confirm or refute these suspicions, however, you will need to see if there is any evidence of alterations in the respiratory and metabolic components of the body's acid-base balance. This entails reviewing the $PaCO_2$ and standard bicarbonate (or base excess), respectively.

Is there evidence of a disturbance in the respiratory component of the body's acid-base balance?

You will remember that the $PaCO_2$ indicates whether there is a disturbance in the respiratory component of the body's acid-base balance.* Take this opportunity therefore to test your memory of what happens to the $PaCO_2$ in the following acid-base disturbances.

- Acute respiratory acidosis
- Chronic respiratory acidosis
- Acute metabolic acidosis
- Chronic metabolic acidosis
- Combined metabolic and respiratory acidosis
- Respiratory alkalosis
- Metabolic alkalosis
- Chronic metabolic alkalosis.

* If this comes as a complete revelation to you, read pages 38–40.

Answers

Acid-base disturbance	Alteration in $PaCO_2$ (normal range 35–45 mm Hg (4·7–6·0 kPa))
Acute respiratory acidosis	Rises (see page 66)
Chronic respiratory acidosis	Rises (see page 73)
Acute metabolic acidosis	Initially unchanged, then falls due to respiratory compensation (see page 77)
Chronic metabolic acidosis	Rises back towards normal if metabolic compensation is effective (see page 82)
Combined metabolic and respiratory acidosis	Rises (see page 84)
Respiratory alkalosis	Fall (see page 93)
Metabolic alkalosis	Initially unchanged, then rises due to respiratory compensation (see page 102)
Chronic metabolic alkalosis	Falls back towards normal if metabolic compensation is effective (see page 105)

With the knowledge of how the $PaCO_2$ has changed, you can then refer back to the pH and consider whether they tally with one another. For example, if the pH was low (that is, the patient had an acidaemia) and the $PaCO_2$ result was high this would indicate that at least part of the acidaemia was due to the respiratory acidosis. Alternatively, if both the pH and $PaCO_2$ were low then the fall in the pH is not a result of the respiratory component of the body's acid-base balance. If it was then the $PaCO_2$ should be high. Consequently, in the last example, the body is either compensating

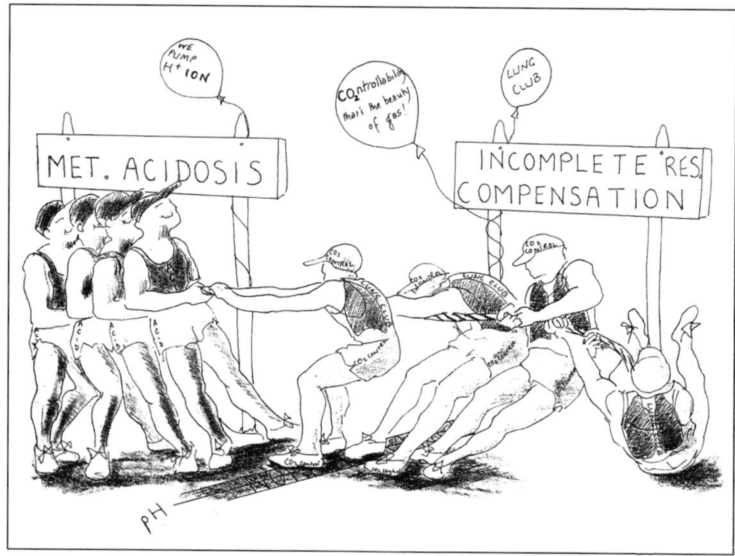

Figure 7.5 Metabolic acidosis *v* respiratory compensation.

incompletely for a metabolic acidosis (figure 7.5) or there is a coexisting primary respiratory alkalosis. In this case, the metabolic acidosis is having a bigger effect on the pH than the respiratory alkalosis (figure 7.6).

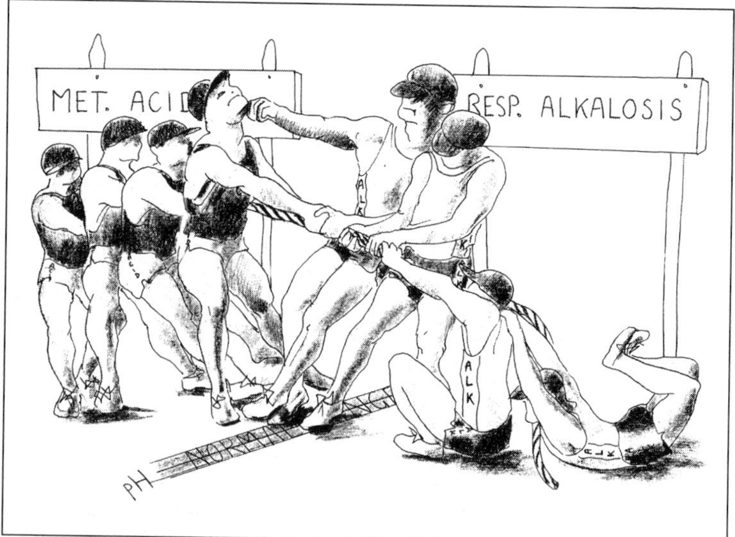

Figure 7.6 Respiratory alkalosis *v* metabolic acidosis.

These points can be summarised in the following table. To test your comprehension take the opportunity to fill in the remaining blank spaces.

pH	$PaCO_2$	Interpretation
Low	High	Acidaemia, part of which is due to a primary respiratory acidosis
Low	Low	Acidaemia from a primary metabolic acidosis in addition to either incomplete respiratory compensation or a primary respiratory alkalosis
High	Low	
High	High	
Normal	High	
Normal	Low	

Answers

pH	$PaCO_2$	Interpretation
Low	High	Acidaemia part of which is due to a primary respiratory acidosis
Low	Low	Acidaemia from a primary metabolic acidosis in addition to either incomplete respiratory compensation or a primary respiratory alkalosis
High	Low	Alkalaemia, part of which at least is due to a primary respiratory alkalosis (see page 94)
High	High	Alkalaemia from a primary metabolic alkalosis in addition to either incomplete respiratory compensation or a primary respiratory acidosis (see page 103)

Normal	**High**	**Primary respiratory acidosis. Either the changes are too small to alter the pH or there is full metabolic compensaton. Alternatively, there is more than one acid-base disturbance and they are cancelling out one another's pH changes (see page 121)**
Normal	**Low**	**Primary respiratory alkalosis. Either the changes are too small to alter the pH or there is full metabolic compensation. Alternatively, there is more than one acid-base disturbance and they are cancelling out one another's pH changes (see page 121)**

To gain further information on whether the respiratory disturbance is the primary acid-base problem, or simply compensatory to a metabolic disturbance, you now need to consider the standard bicarbonate and base excess concentrations.

Is there evidence of a disturbance in the metabolic component of the body's acid base balance?

We have described previously that both the standard bicarbonate and base excess concentrations indicate whether there is a disturbance in the metabolic component of the body's acid-base balance.* If you are happy with this concept take this opportunity to test your memory further by describing what happens to these concentrations in the following acid-base disturbances.

Acid-base disturbance	**Alteration in standard HCO_3^- concentration (normal range 21–27 mmol/l) or base excess (normal range ±2 mmol/l)**
Acute respiratory acidosis	
Chronic respiratory acidosis	

* If you want to refresh your understanding of this point, read pages 33–4.

Acute metabolic acidosis	
Combined metabolic and respiratory acidosis	
Respiratory alkalosis	
Metabolic alkalosis	

Answers

Acid-base disturbance	Alteration in standard HCO_3^- concentration (normal range 21–27 mmol/l) or base excess (normal range ±2 mmol/l)
Acute respiratory acidosis	**Initially unchanged, then rises due to compensation (see page 66)**
Chronic respiratory acidosis	**Rises (see page 73)**
Acute metabolic acidosis	**Falls (see page 77)**
Combined metabolic and respiratory acidosis	**Falls (see page 84)**
Respiratory alkalosis	**Initially unchanged, then falls due to compensation (see page 95)**
Metabolic alkalosis	**Rises (see page 102)**

With the knowledge of how the standard bicarbonate and base excess concentrations have altered you can now review the conclusion drawn from the pH and $PaCO_2$ result. For example, consider the case where the pH is low and the $PaCO_2$, standard bicarbonate, and base excess concentrations are all high. The most likely reason for this is a respiratory acidosis that has persisted long enough to enable some metabolic compensation to occur (figure 7.7). A less common cause would be a respiratory acidosis and combined metabolic alkalosis. For this to be true the respiratory acidosis would have to be producing a bigger effect on the pH than the metabolic alkalosis because of the overall acidaemia (figure 7.8).

These points can be summarised in the following table. To test

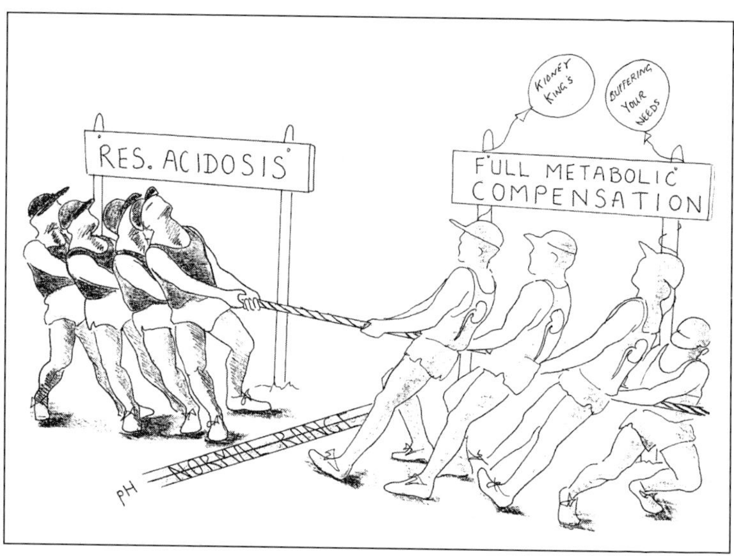

Figure 7.7 Respiratory acidosis *v* full metabolic compensation.

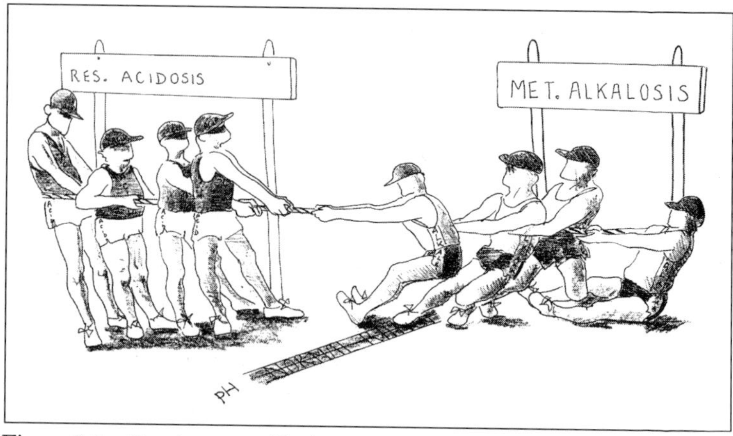

Figure 7.8 Respiratory acidosis *v* metabolic alkalosis.

your comprehension take the opportunity to fill in the blank spaces (answers follow).

pH	$PaCO_2$	Standard HCO_3^- and base excess	Interpretation
Low	High	High	Acidaemia from either a primary respiratory acidosis with incomplete metabolic compensation or primary respiratory acidosis and primary metabolic alkalosis (see pages 66–76 and 99–107)
Low	High	Low	
Low	Low	Low	
High	Low	High	
High	Low	Low	
High	High	High	
Normal	High	High	
Normal	Low	Low	

Answers

pH	$PaCO_2$	Standard HCO_3^- and base excess	Interpretation
Low	High	High	Acidaemia from either a primary respiratory acidosis with incomplete metabolic compensation or respiratory acidosis with a primary metabolic alkalosis (see pages 66–76 and 99–107)

Low	**High**	**Low**	**Acidaemia from a combined primary respiratory and metabolic acidosis (see page 89)**
Low	**Low**	**Low**	**Acidaemia from either a primary metabolic acidosis with incomplete respiratory compensation or a primary metabolic acidosis with a primary respiratory alkalosis (see pages 77–82)**
High	**Low**	**High**	**Alkalaemia from a combined primary respiratory and metabolic alkalosis (this is very rare)***
High	**Low**	**Low**	**Alkalaemia from either a primary respiratory alkalosis with incomplete metabolic compensation or a primary respiratory alkalosis with a primary metabolic acidosis (see pages 94–8)**
High	**High**	**High**	**Alkalaemia from either a primary metabolic alkalosis with incomplete respiratory compensation or primary metabolic alkalosis with a primary respiratory acidosis (see pages 102–4)**
Normal	**High**	**High**	**Combined respiratory acidosis and metabolic alkalosis that are cancelling out one another's pH changes. These could both be primary disturbances or one could be completely compensating for the other (see pages 73 and 121)**

* This is one to keep for your personal collection because it is a very rare combination.

Normal	**Low**	**Low**	**Combined respiratory alkalosis and metabolic acidosis that are cancelling out one another's pH changes. These could both be primary disturbances or one could be completely compensating for the other (see pages 98–9, 82–4, and 121)**

As you will see, there may be more than one possible answer. To decide which is the correct one, we need to examine the data in more detail.

Is there a single or multiple acid-base disturbance?

With time, a disturbance in one part of the body's acid-base system will give rise to compensatory changes. In longstanding cases, therefore, the $PaCO_2$, standard bicarbonate, and base excess will probably be outside their normal ranges. This can make it difficult to determine if the underlying problem is in the respiratory or metabolic systems. A helpful rule in this situation is to see which is the most abnormal parameter because this is usually the one with the primary problem. In applying this, however, it is important to be aware that the body can have more than one acid-base abnormality. For example, patients suffering from a cardiac arrest will have a combined respiratory and metabolic acidosis.

> **Halt: Key point**
>
> **The underlying acid-base abnormality is usually in the system that is furthest from the normal range**

To determine whether a single or multiple acid-base disturbance is present we need to consider how much the $PaCO_2$, actual bicarbonate, and base excess have changed. If these concentrations fall within certain limits then there is usually only a single acid-base disturbance, with or without compensation. Alternatively, if they are outside this range then the patient probably has more than one acid-base disturbance.

Below we describe two methods of assessing these changes. As both systems work, it is entirely up to you to choose the one you prefer. For those who like looking at pictures we would recommend

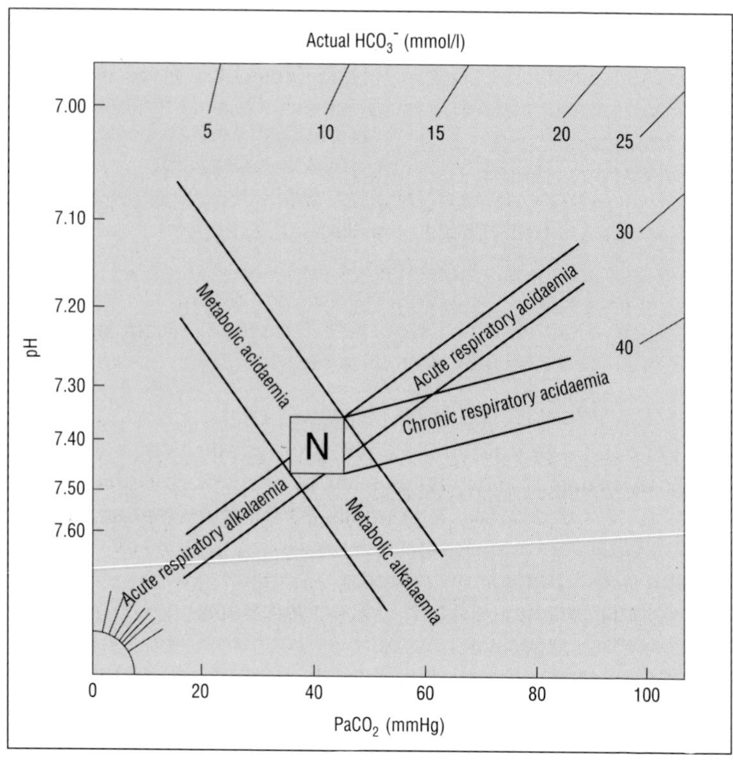

Figure 7.9 The possible ranges associated with various acid base disturbances.

using a graph. Alternatively, for those who prefer to do mental arithmetic, we would recommend the memorising of certain numbers.

Graphical method

You will recognise figure 7.9 because it was gradually built up over chapters 5 and 6. Take a moment to familiarise yourself with its layout and what it is showing. In particular note:

- The graph is showing how the pH alters with changes in $PaCO_2$.
- Cutting diagonally across the graph are lines that indicate the concentration of actual bicarbonate. These are known as isopleths.
- As the concentration of bicarbonate increases the gradients of the isopleths fall—that is, the lines become less steep.

- The square box indicates the normal range for pH, $PaCO_2$, and actual bicarbonate concentration.
- Fanning out from this box are the possible ranges of normal compensatory responses you could expect with single acid-base disturbances.
- The bands representing the acute respiratory disturbances run about parallel to the isopleths. In other words acute respiratory acidosis and alkalosis will alter the pH and $PaCO_2$ but will have little effect on the bicarbonate concentration. These bands do not include patients who have had long enough to develop compensation and so alter their bicarbonate concentrations. Instead, these patients are represented in the chronic respiratory acidosis group.
- The band representing the metabolic disturbances runs across the isopleths. Therefore metabolic acidosis and alkalosis will alter the bicarbonate concentration as well as the pH and $PaCO_2$. These bands include patients who are using respiratory compensation to counteract the pH changes. They do not, however, include those patients who have had long enough to develop metabolic compensation (that is, those who have a chronic metabolic disturbance).

By using this graph you can plot the results from the blood gas analysis (figure 7.10). If the results lie within one of the broad bands shown, then there is probably only one acid-base disturbance, with or without compensation. If the results lie outside these normal ranges, however, then there is probably more than one acid-base disturbance. To practice applying these concepts, plot the following values and interpret the result.

pH	$PaCO_2$	Actual bicarbonate	Interpretation
7·53	30	25	
7·22	23	9	
7·41	37	24	
7·28	58	26·5	
7·60	51	49	
7·38	72	40	
7·11	58	18	
7·41	21	13	
7·64	30	32	
7·47	64	45	

Figure 7.10 shows the plotting of the values and the table below lists the interpetation of the results.

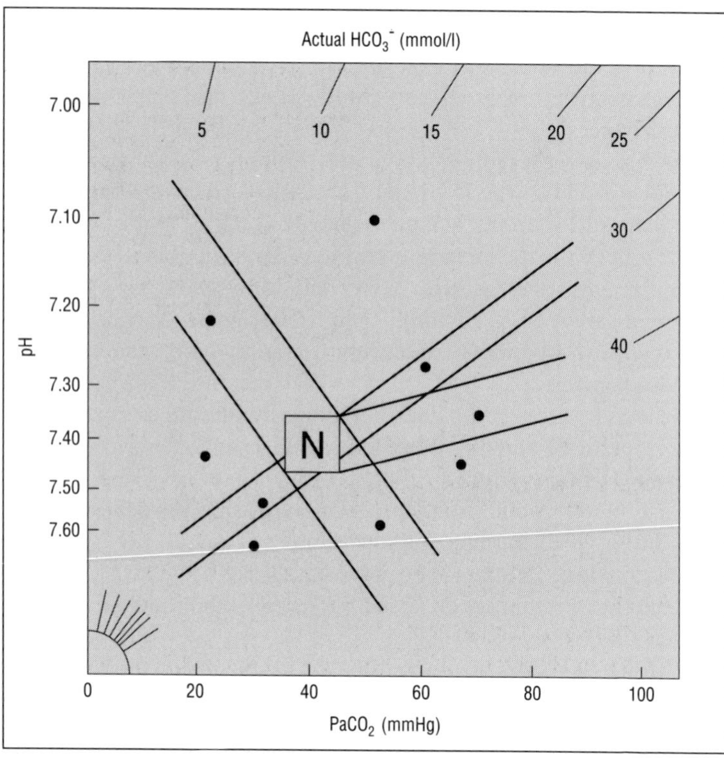

Figure 7.10 Results of examples plotted on graph.

pH	$PaCO_2$	Actual bicarbonate	Interpretation
7·53	30	25	Alkalaemia due to an acute respiratory alkalosis
7·22	23	9	Acidaemia due to a metabolic acidosis
7·41	37	24	Normal
7·28	58	26·5	Acidaemia due to an acute respiratory acidosis
7·60	51	49	Alkalaemia due to a metabolic alkalosis
7·38	72	40	Chronic respiratory acidosis with full metabolic compensation
7·11	58	18	Acidaemia due to a respiratory and metabolic acidosis
7·41	21	13	Combined respiratory alkalosis and metabolic acidosis. These could both be primary disturbances or there may be a chronic primary respiratory alkalosis with full metabolic compensation

pH	$PaCO_2$	Actual bicarbonate	Interpretation
7·64	30	32	Alkalaemia due to a respiratory and metabolic alkalosis
7·47	64	45	Combined respiratory acidosis and metabolic alkalosis. These are both likely to be primary disturbances. (A useful rule of thumb is that a plasma standard bicarbonate concentration $\geqslant 40$ mmol/l indicates that there is some degree of primary metabolic acidosis. It is rare for the body to achieve this level as part of a metabolic compensation to a respiratory acidosis)

Box 7.8 Expected changes*

Acute respiratory acidosis (the last two digits of the pH should be the same as the value for $PaCO_2$—for example, a pH of 7·30 should be accompanied by a $PaCO_2$ of 30 mm Hg):

- A 1·0 mm Hg rise in $PaCO_2$ produces a 0·1 mmol/l rise in actual HCO_3^-

Chronic respiratory acidosis:

- A 1·0 mm Hg rise in $PaCO_2$ produces a 0·4 mmol/l rise in actual HCO_3^-

Acute respiratory alkalosis:

- A 1·0 mm Hg fall in $PaCO_2$ produces a 0·2 mmol/l fall in actual HCO_3^-

Chronic respiratory alkalosis:

- A 1·0 mm Hg fall in $PaCO_2$ produces a 0·5 mmol/l fall in actual HCO_3^-

Metabolic acidosis:

- A 1·0 mmol/l fall in actual HCO_3^- produces a 1·0–1·3 mm Hg fall in $PaCO_2$

Metabolic alkalosis:

- A 1 mmol/l rise in actual HCO_3^- produces a 0·6 mm Hg rise in $PaCO_2$

* All these values are taken from the middle of the normal ranges—for instance 40 mm Hg (5·3 kPa) for the $PaCO_2$ and 24·5 mmol/l for the actual bicarbonate concentration

Arithmetic method

This system has the disadvantage of using the older units for $PaCO_2$—that is, mm Hg. Nevertheless, by applying the numbers listed in box 7.8 you will be able to determine if the changes in $PaCO_2$ and actual bicarbonate are appropriate for a single acid-base disturbance.*

If there is an inconsistency between analysis of the blood sample and the results derived by calculation then the patient probably has more than one acid-base disturbance.

With these numbers practice with the following examples (answers follow).

1. In acute respiratory acidosis, what actual HCO_3^- concentration would you expect to find if the patient's $PaCO_2$ was:

$PaCO_2$ (mm Hg)	Calculation	Actual HCO_3^- (mmol/l)
49	24·5 + (9 × 0·1)	25·4
60		
73		

2 In chronic respiratory acidosis, what actual HCO_3^- concentration would you expect to find if the patient's $PaCO_2$ was:

$PaCO_2$ (mm Hg)	Calculation	Actual HCO_3^- (mmol/l)
50	24·5 + (10 × 0·4)	28·0
65		
58		

3 In acute respiratory alkalosis, what actual HCO_3^- concentration would you expect to find if the patient's $PaCO_2$ was:

$PaCO_2$ (mm Hg)	Calculation	Actual HCO_3^- (mmol/l)
30	24·5 − (10 × 0·2)	22·5
28		
20		

* These calculations give you the *actual* concentration because they are reflecting the respiratory and metabolic components of the body's acid-base balance. By definition, the standard bicarbonate concentration reflects only the metabolic aspects.

4 In chronic respiratory alkalosis, what actual HCO_3^- concentration would you expect to find if the patient's $PaCO_2$ was:

$PaCO_2$ (mm Hg)	Calculation	Actual HCO_3^- (mmol/l)
32	24·5 – (8 × 0·5)	20·5
29		
26		

5 In metabolic acidosis, what $PaCO_2$ concentration would you expect to find if the patient's HCO_3^- was:

Actual HCO_3^- (mmol/l)	Calculation	$PaCO_2$ (mm Hg)
12	(40 – (1·3 × 12)) – (40 – (1 × 12))	24·4 – 28·0
16		
18		

6 In metabolic alkalosis, what $PaCO_2$ concentration would you expect to find if the patient's HCO_3^- was:

Actual HCO_3^- (mmol/l)	Calculation	$PaCO_2$ (mm Hg)
32·5	40 + (0·6 × 8)	44·8
34·5		
37·5		

Answers

Question 1

$PaCO_2$ (mm Hg)	Calculation	Actual HCO_3^- (mmol/l)
49	24·5 + (9 × 0·1)	25·4
60	24·5 + (20 × 0·1)	26·5
73	24·5 + (33 × 0·1)	27·8

Question 2

$PaCO_2$ (mm Hg)	Calculation	Actual HCO_3^- (mmol/l)
50	24·5 + (10 × 0·4)	28·5
65	24·5 + (25 × 0·4)	34·5
58	24·5 + (18 × 0·4]	31·7

Question 3

$PaCO_2$ (mm Hg)	Calculation	Actual HCO_3^- (mmol/l)
30	24·5 − (10 × 0·2)	22·5
28	24·5 − (12 × 0·2)	22·1
20	24·5 − (20 × 0·2)	20·5

Question 4

$PaCO_2$ (mm Hg)	Calculation	Actual HCO_3^- (mmol/l)
32	24·5 − (8 × 0·5)	20·0
29	24·5 − (11 × 0·5)	18·5
26	24·5 − (14 × 0·5)	17·0

Question 5

Actual HCO_3^- (mmol/l)	Calculation	$PaCO_2$ (mm Hg)
12·5	(40 − (1·3 × 12)) − (40 − (1 × 12))	24·4 − 28·0
16·5	(40 − (1·3 × 9)) − (40 − (1 × 9))	28·3 − 31·0
18·5	(40 − (1·3 × 6)) − (40 − (1 × 6))	32·2 − 34·0

Question 6

Actual HCO_3^- (mmol/l)	Calculation	$PaCO_2$ (mm Hg)
32·5	40 + (0·6 × 8)	44·8
34·5	40 + (0·6 × 10)	46·0
37·5	40 + (0·6 × 13)	47·8

You have now finished the interpretation of the parameters in the blood gas analysis that provide information on the patient's acid-base balance. The final value that needs to be assessed in an arterial sample is the partial pressure of oxygen. This is important because a failure to take up oxygen can lead to many adverse conditions, including hypoxia. With regard to the acid-base balance, hypoxia can give rise to metabolic acidosis because it causes the cells to change to anaerobic metabolism and so produce excessive quantities of lactic acid (see page 82). In addition, the PaO_2 also gives an indication of respiratory function, which may add further clues when you analyse the $PaCO_2$.

Is there any defect in oxygen uptake?

A PaO_2 on its own will not allow you to answer this question because this value depends on the inspired concentration of oxygen (FIO_2) (see pages 51–3). By knowing the FIO_2, however, it is possible to have a rough idea of what the PaO_2 should be if the patient is ventilating normally.

As atmospheric pressure is 760 mm Hg (about 100 kPa), 1% of this value is 7·6 mm Hg (about 1 kPa). This would mean that inspiring 30% O_2 from a face mask would produce an inspired partial pressure of oxygen of 228 mm Hg or 30 kPa. This should lead to a PaO_2 of around 170 mm Hg (22 kPa) because there is normally a drop of about 60 mm Hg (8 kPa) between the partial pressure of oxygen inspired at the mouth and that in the arterial system. With age, however, this can increase to around 75 mm Hg (10 kPa).

Halt: Key point

As a rule of thumb a difference between the inspired oxygen concentration and the PaO_2 of greater than 75 mm Hg (10 kPa) would imply that there is a defect in the uptake of oxygen

For example, an arterial PaO_2 of 250 mm Hg (33·3 kPa) in a patient breathing 40% oxygen is within normal limits. In contrast, a PaO_2 of 180 mm Hg (24·0 kPa) in a patient breathing 50% oxygen indicates that there is a defect in the take up of oxygen because the expected value is as follows.

In mm Hg—An inspired oxygen of 50% will have a partial pressure of $50 \times 760/100 = 380$ mm Hg (that is, half the normal atmospheric pressure). This would mean the expected PaO_2 would be at least $380 - 75 = 305$ mm Hg.

In kPa—An inspired oxygen of 50% will have a partial pressure of about 50 kPa. This would mean the expected PaO_2 would be at least $50 - 10 = 40$ kPa.

Try out your understanding of this concept with the following imaginary cases:

PaO_2	FIO_2 (%)	Interpretation
90 mm Hg (12·0 kPa)	0·2 (21%)	
150 mm Hg (20·0 kPa)	0·4 (40%)	
100 mm Hg (13·3 kPa)	1·0 (100%)	
200 mm Hg (26·7 kPa)	0·85 (85%)	
110 mm Hg (14·7 kPa)	0·3 (30%)	

Answers

PaO_2	FIO_2 (%)	Interpretation
90 mm Hg (12·0 kPa)	0·2 (21%)	Within normal limits
150 mm Hg (20·0 kPa)	0·4 (40%)	Defect in O_2 uptake
100 mm Hg (13·3 kPa)	1·0 (100%)	Defect in O_2 uptake
200 mm Hg (26·7 kPa)	0·85 (85%)	Defect in O_2 uptake
110 mm Hg (14·7 kPa)	0·3 (30%)	Defect in O_2 uptake

Integration of clinical findings and data interpretation

You are now on the final leg of your interpretation of the blood gas results. What remains is to compare your clinical suspicions with the data analysis. The following options are possible:

Clinical suspicion	Data interpretation	Conclusion
Single acid-base disturbance	Single acid-base disturbance	Single acid-base disturbance
Multiple acid-base disturbance	Multiple acid-base disturbance	Multiple acid-base disturbance
Multiple acid-base disturbance	Single acid-base disturbance	Either cause of acid-base disturbance is too early or too mild to produce biochemical change, or error in clinical assessment or in data interpretation
Single acid-base disturbance	Multiple acid-base disturbance	Error in clinical assessment or in data interpretation

To test this system properly it is best to see how it works on some clinical cases. Firstly, take a moment to remind yourself of the questions which you need to ask:

History

- Are any symptoms due to the cause of an acid-base disturbance?
- Are any symptoms as a result of an acid-base disturbance?

Data

- Is the pH abnormal?
- Is the $PaCO_2$ abnormal?
- Are the standard bicarbonate and base excess concentrations abnormal?
- Is there a single or multiple acid-base disturbance?
- Is the PaO_2 uptake abnormal?

Integration

- Do the suspicions from the history agree with the data analysis?

Example 1

History—A 17 year old schoolgirl who was normally in good health was found at home by her parents in a restless and confused state. She was pale, sweaty, and hyperventilating.

Results—While she was breathing room air, an arterial sample was taken for blood gas analysis. The results were:

Measure	Normal	Patient
pH	7·36–7·44	7·10
$PaCO_2$	35–45 mm Hg (4·7–6·0 kPa)	18 mm Hg (2·4 kPa)
Actual HCO_3^-	21–28 mmol/l	6 mmol/l
Standard HCO_3^-	21–27 mmol/l	10 mmol/l
Base excess	±2 mmol/l	−14 mmol/l
PaO_2	Over 90 mm Hg (12·0 kPa) on room air	105 mm Hg (14 kPa)

Analysis

History—The hyperventilation may be a primary problem (such as anxiety) or compensation for an underlying metabolic acidosis. You would therefore suspect from the history that there could be either a respiratory alkalosis or a metabolic acidosis with respiratory compensation. With regard to acid-base balance you can also deduce from the history that this is an acute event. It is therefore unlikely that there would be sufficient time for any metabolic compensation in either of the possible acid-base disturbances suspected.

Systematic analysis of the blood gas results

Is there an acidaemia or alkalaemia?—As the pH is below 7·36, there is an acidaemia.

Is there evidence of a disturbance in the respiratory component of the body's acid-base balance?—Yes, the $PaCO_2$ is low. In the light of the pH this indicates that there is either respiratory compensation to a metabolic acidosis or a combination of a big metabolic acidosis and smaller primary respiratory alkalosis.

Is there evidence of a disturbance in the metabolic component of the body's acid-base balance?—Yes, the standard bicarbonate concentration is low, and the base excess is very negative. In the light of the pH and $PaCO_2$ this supports the two possibilities suggested above.

Is there a single or multiple acid-base disturbance?—By using the graph in figure 7.9 (page 132), you can see that the results lie within the metabolic acidosis band. This would imply that the patient has a metabolic acidosis with respiratory compensation and has not had time to develop metabolic compensation.

By using the arithmetic model if the patient had a metabolic acidosis, as a 1 mmol/l fall in actual HCO_3^- produces a 1·0–1·3 mm Hg fall in $PaCO_2$, an 18·5 mmol/l fall in HCO_3^- would produce an 18·5–24·1 mm Hg fall in $PaCO_2$. Therefore if we use the midpoints of the normal ranges, this patient's $PaCO_2$ should be between:

$$(40-18{\cdot}5) \text{ and } (40-24{\cdot}1) = 15{\cdot}9-21{\cdot}5 \text{ mm Hg}$$

As this incorporates the level in the arterial blood sample, this patient probably has a single acid-base disturbance that is a metabolic acidosis.

Is the PaO_2 uptake abnormal?—The expected PaO_2 when a patient is breathing room air is over 90 mm Hg (over 12·0 kPa). There is therefore no evidence of any problem in oxygen uptake in this patient.

Integrate the clinical findings with the data interpretation

The clinical and data analyses tally. This girl has a metabolic acidosis with respiratory compensation. Your next move would be to determine what is the cause of the acidosis. This entails carrying out further tests that are selected in the light of the patient's history and physical examination. A list of common causes of metabolic acidosis is given on page 76. The most likely cause in this case is either an overdose or diabetic ketoacidosis.

A metabolic acidosis was chosen first partly because of the history and partly because of a rule of thumb which states that:

> "when the $PaCO_2$, standard bicarbonate, and base excess concentrations are abnormal, the one that most closely corresponds to the pH and deviates most from normal is probably the one causing the biggest effect on the pH".

Consequently the metabolic component of the body's acid-base balance was suspected as being the primary problem in this patient. Obviously if the subsequent calculations did not work out then the other possibilities would be explored.

Example 2

History—A 30 year old woman attempted to commit suicide by throwing herself into a canal having taken an overdose of alcohol. Fortunately she was saved by a passing policeman and brought to the emergency department. On examination she was pale, cold, and confused. Her tympanic temperature was 28·4°C, and she had a respiratory rate of 18/min. Her heart rate was 107/min and blood pressure 137/90 mm Hg. Auscultation of her chest revealed bilateral expiratory rhonchi and crepitations.

Results—While the patient was breathing 85% oxygen by a non-rebreathing mask with a reservoir, an arterial sample was taken for blood gas analysis. The results were:

Measure	Normal	Patient
pH	7·36–7·44	7·23
$PaCO_2$	35–45 mm Hg (4·7–6·0 kPa)	41·5 mm Hg (5·3 kPa)
Actual HCO_3^-	21–28 mmol/l	16·7 mmol/l
Standard HCO_3^-	21–27 mmol/l	16·4 mmol/l
Base excess	±2 mmol/l	−10·2 mmol/l
PaO_2	Over 90 mm Hg (12·0 kPa) on room air	86·0 mm Hg (11·5 kPa)

Analysis

History—In situations of near drowning, patients can aspirate water and impair their oxygen uptake. This can lead to both tissue hypoxia as well as carbon dioxide retention. This woman is at risk therefore of developing a combined respiratory and metabolic acidosis. She could also have developed a metabolic acidosis secondary to the alcohol ingestion as well as the reduced tissue perfusion after the hypothermia.

Depending on the state of her lungs, she may or may not be able to mount a respiratory compensation to the metabolic acidosis. If she has, then you would expect her $PaCO_2$ level to be below the normal range.

Systematic analysis of the blood gas results

Is there an acidaemia or alkalaemia?—The pH is low therefore there is an acidaemia.

Is there evidence of a disturbance in the respiratory component of the body's acid-base balance?—The $PaCO_2$ is within the normal range. This could mean there is no respiratory disturbance. As the pH is abnormal, however, this is unlikely because you would expect the $PaCO_2$ to be either above (that is, causing the acidosis) or below (that is, responding to the acidosis) the normal range. A more likely explanation is that the patient is changing from a state of carbon dioxide retention to one of increased carbon dioxide removal. This would come about when the patient was transferred from the water to the resuscitation room and given a high inspired oxygen concentration.

Is there evidence of a disturbance in the metabolic component of the body's acid-base balance?—Yes, the standard bicarbonate and base excess are lowered, indicating a metabolic acidosis. In the light of the pH this means the patient has at least a metabolic acidosis.

Is there a single or multiple acid-base disturbance?—This patient has a combined respiratory and metabolic acidosis.

By using the graph in figure 7.9 (page 132) you can see that the results lie between the standard bands for metabolic and acute respiratory acidosis. This implies that more than one acid-base disturbance is present.

By using the arithmetic model, if the patient had only an acute metabolic acidosis then the expected $PaCO_2$ varies between:

$$(40(1{\cdot}0 \times (24{\cdot}5 - 16{\cdot}7))) \text{ and } (40 - (1{\cdot}3 \times (24{\cdot}5 - 16{\cdot}7)))$$

$29{\cdot}9 - 32{\cdot}2(3{\cdot}9 - 4{\cdot}2$ kPa)

As the patient's $PaCO_2$ lies above this range, a primary metabolic acidosis cannot fully explain the carbon dioxide concentration. Consequently, there has to be a coexisting respiratory acidosis giving rise to the additional carbon dioxide.

Is the PaO_2 abnormal?—By using mm Hg an inspired oxygen of 85% will have a partial pressure of $85 \times 760/100 = 646$ mm Hg. This would mean the expected PaO_2 would be at least $646 - 76 = 570$ mm Hg.

By using kPa an inspired oxygen of 85% will have a partial pressure of approximately 85 kPa. This would mean the expected PaO_2 would be at least $85 - 10 = 75$ kPa. As the patient's PaO_2 is much lower than expected there is an impaired oxygen uptake.

Integrate the clinical findings with the data interpretation

The clinical and data analyses tally. This woman has a combined respiratory and metabolic acidosis with impaired oxygen uptake. Before resuscitation her $PaCO_2$ was probably above the normal range. After the clearing of her airway and the administration of oxygen, however, she has begun to develop respiratory compensation for her metabolic acidosis. As a result the $PaCO_2$ has fallen to lie within the normal range. After a further half hour of resuscitation her $PaCO_2$ fell below the normal range as the respiratory compensation increased.

Summary

Analysis of a blood gas result begins by assessing the patient clinically and studying their medical notes. By doing this you will learn what the medical problems are and how they are being treated. With this information you can then interpret the blood gas result appropriately by using the system described in box 7.9. In contrast, simply using the laboratory results in isolation increases the chances of missing a coexisting acid-base disturbance.

Quiz

This chapter has discussed how to interpret the blood gas results. It has been a long chapter and has summarised much of what has been said in previous chapters. It is therefore very important that you take a well earned rest. When you have recuperated, consider

Box 7.9 A system for interpreting blood gas results

History

- Any symptoms due to the cause of an acid-base disturbance?
- Any symptoms as a result of an acid-base disturbance?

Data

- Is the pH abnormal?
- Is the $PaCO_2$ abnormal?
- Is the standard bicarbonate (base excess) concentration abnormal?
- Is there a single or multiple acid-base disturbance?
- Is the PaO_2 abnormal?

Integration

- Do the suspicions from the history agree with the data analysis?

what you have read before testing your comprehension with quiz 7 below.

Quiz 7 (answers on page 157–67)

1 **What effect does an increase in $PaCO_2$ have on consciousness?**

2 **How does the concentration of potassium ions change when there are alterations in the concentration of hydrogen ions in the extracellular fluid?**

3 **Why does a mild metabolic acidosis give rise to cold and clammy skin?**

4 **What level of compensation is usually present in acute, single acid-base disturbances?**

5 **Name three reasons why the pH may be normal?**

6 **What is your assessment of the acid-base disturbance in the following clinical example?**

History—A 65 year old woman was brought to the department with a two day history of increasing shortness of breath and cough. She was known to suffer from chronic obstructive pulmonary disease (COPD).

Results—While the patient was breathing 30% oxygen via a mask, an arterial sample was taken for blood gas analysis. The results were:

Measure	Normal	Patient
pH	7·36–7·44	7·32
$PaCO_2$	35–45 mm Hg (4·7–6·0 kPa)	63·2 mm Hg (8·4 kPa)
Actual HCO_3^-	21–28 mmol/l	29·8 mmol/l
Standard HCO_3^-	21–27 mmol/l	31·6 mmol/l
Base excess	±2 mmol/l	3·5 mmol/l
PaO_2	Over 90 mm Hg (12·0 kPa) on room air	86·8 mm Hg (11·6 kPa)

7 What is your assessment of the acid-base disturbance in the following clinical example?

History—A 42 year old man was brought to the emergency department having taken an overdose of dopthiepin one hour previously. In transit to hospital he had a generalised epileptic fit. He became unconscious and was breathing spontaneously at 7 breaths/min.

Results—While the patient was receiving 85% oxygen by a non-rebreathing mask with a reservoir bag, an arterial sample was taken for blood gas analysis. The results were:

Measure	Normal	Patient
pH	7·36–7·44	6·71
$PaCO_2$	35–45 mm Hg (4·7–6·0 kPa)	87·9 mm Hg (11·7 kPa)
Actual HCO_3^-	21–28 mmol/l	10·5 mmol/l
Standard HCO_3^-	21–27 mmol/l	4·7 mmol/l
Base excess	±2 mmol/l	−22·4 mmol
PaO_2	Over 90 mm Hg (12·0 kPa) on room air	250·2 mm Hg (33·4 kPa)

8 What is your assessment of the acid-base disturbance in the following clinical example?

History—A 35 year old man was brought to the department. He was known to have insulin dependent diabetes and had a three day history of fever, cough, and shortness of breath.

Results—While the patient was receiving room air, an arterial sample was taken for blood gas analysis. The results were:

Measure	Normal	Patient
pH	7·36–7·44	7·36
$PaCO_2$	35–45 mm Hg (4·7–6·0 kPa)	22·7 mm Hg (3·0 kPa)
Actual HCO_3^-	21–28 mmol/l	15·1 mmol/l
Standard HCO_3^-	21–27 mmol/l	12·6 mmol/l
Base excess	2 mmol/l	−10·7 mmol/l
PaO_2	Over 90 mm Hg (12·0 kPa) on room air	80·5 mm Hg (10·7 kPa)

9. What is your assessment of the acid-base disturbance in the following clinical example?

History—A 64 year old previously healthy woman had a cardiac arrest at home. Her husband witnessed the collapse and started cardiopulmonary resuscitation as soon as he had phoned for an ambulance. The paramedics arrived within 5 minutes and diagnosed ventricular fibrillation. After the sixth shock the patient regained a palpable sinus beat of 70/min but did not breathe spontaneously. On arrival at hospital she was intubated and ventilated at 15 breaths/min. She was unconscious but had a heart rate of 80 beats/min and a blood pressure of 100/60 mm Hg.

Results—While the patient was breathing 100% oxygen via an endotracheal tube, an arterial sample was taken for blood gas analysis. The results were:

Measure	Normal	Patient
pH	7·36–7·44	7·44
$PaCO_2$	35–45 mm Hg (4·7–6·0 kPa)	15·9 mm Hg (2·12 kPa)
Actual HCO_3^-	21–28 mmol/l	10·7 mmol/l
Standard HCO_3^-	21–27 mmol/l	15·9 mmol/l
Base excess	±2 mmol/l	−12·8 mmol/l
PaO_2	Over 90 mm Hg (12·0 kPa) on room air	636·1 mm Hg (84·8 kPa)

10 What is your assessment of the acid-base disturbance in the following clinical example?

History—An 80 year old woman had a partial colectomy for carcinoma of the sigmoid four days previously. Postoperatively a nasogastric tube had been inserted because she was vomiting. This was draining about 2 l of gastric fluid a day.

Results—While the patient was breathing 45% oxygen via a mask, an arterial sample was taken for blood gas analysis. The results were:

Measure	Normal	Patient
pH	7·36–7·44	7·56
$PaCO_2$	35–45 mm Hg (4·7–6·0 kPa)	38·2 mm Hg (5·1 kPa)
Actual HCO_3^-	21–28 mmol/l	34·0 mmol/l
Standard HCO_3^-	21–27 mmol/l	34·8 mmol/l
Base excess	±2 mmol/l	+12·2 mmol/l
PaO_2	Over 90 mm Hg (12·0 kPa) on room air	143 mm Hg (19·1 kPa)

Answers to end of chapter quizzes

Quiz 1

1 Radial, brachial, and femoral (see pages 2–4). The radial artery lies closest to the skin surface (see page 2).
2 Impaired distal circulation, underlying skeletal trauma, and the presence of an arteriovenous fistula (see page 2).
3 The femoral vein (see page 4).
4 To stop the sample clotting and therefore invalidating the assessment by the blood gas analyser (see page 4).
5 It makes it acidotic (see page 4).
6 30° for the brachial artery and 70° for the femoral artery (see page 8).
7 Sluggish filling of the syringe (see page 10). You cannot rely on the colour of blood as it may be dark because of the patient having a low concentration of oxygen in his or her circulation. Further clues will come when you study the blood result, but this must take into account the clinical state of the patient and the inspired concentration of oxygen.
8 5 ml (see page 10).
9 Every day (see page 12).
10 When it will be longer than 5 minutes before the sample can be analysed (see page 6).

Quiz 2

1 0·584 g (584 mg):

1 molar solution = 58·4 g sodium chloride (the gram molecular weight) in 1 litre (see page 16)

$$\text{therefore 10 ml of the solution} = \frac{10 \times 58{\cdot}4}{1000}\ \text{g} = 0{\cdot}584\ \text{g}$$

2 0·2 g (200 mg):

2% lignocaine (lidocaine) = 2 g in 100 ml of saline (see page 16)

$$\text{therefore 10 ml of 2\% lignocaine} = \frac{2 \times 10}{100}\ \text{g} = 0{\cdot}2\ \text{g}$$

3 30·4 mm Hg (4·0 kPa)

The partial pressure of a particular gas in a mixture = percentage volume × total pressure of the gas (see page 18–19)

therefore the PCO_2 in dry air at sea level = 0·04 × 760 = 30·4 mm Hg (4·0 kPa)

4 593·3 mm Hg (78·1 kPa)

The partial pressure of a particular gas is a mixture = percentage volume × total pressure of the gas (see page 19)

therefore the partial pressure of nitrogen in dry air at sea level = 78·06 × 760 = 593·3 mm Hg (78·1 kPa)

5 The partial pressure of oxygen in arterial blood (see page 20).

6 5·3 kPa

1 kPa = 7·5 mm Hg (see page 21)

$$\text{therefore 40 mm Hg} = \frac{40}{7{\cdot}5}\ \text{kPa} = 5{\cdot}3\ \text{kPa}$$

7 An acidaemia means the pH is below the normal range (that is, below 7·36). An acidosis means that there is an underlying process that is producing excess acid. However, there does not necessarily have to be a low pH. That would depend on whether the body was also producing excessive amount of base at the same time (see page 25).

8 A base is a hydrogen ion acceptor. In contrast, an alkali is a substance that donates a type of base known as hydroxide ions (OH^-) (see page 22–3).

9 Examples of intracellular buffers include proteins and organic phosphates. Examples of extracellular buffer include proteins, phosphates, ammonia, and the carbonic acid-bicarbonate system (see pages 26–7).

10 A base of −6 mmol/l means that 6 mmol of a strong base would have to be added to 1 litre of blood to get the pH to 7·4 while it was kept at 37°C and a $PaCO_2$ of 40 mm Hg (see page 34).

Quiz 3

1 No. We normally produce vast quantities of acid each day as a byproduct of the metabolism of the food we have ingested (see page 37).
2 The intracellular and extracellular buffers (see page 37).
3 The normal range of arterial partial pressure of CO_2 in a person breathing room air is 35–45 mm Hg (4·7–6·0 kPa) (see page 20).
4 The normal pH range is 7·36–7·44, and this is 36–44 nmol/l of hydrogen ions (see page 24).
5 21–27 mmol/l (see page 33).
6 Both increase by the same amount (see page 40).
7 The standard bicarbonate concentration falls (see page 41).
8 Red blood cells and renal tubular cells (it is also found in large quantities in the gastric mucosa because it is used in the production of hydrochloric acid).
9 The respiratory component responds to the metabolic defect by altering the amount of carbon dioxide removed from the body (see page 45).
10 The metabolic component responds to the respiratory defect by altering the amount of bicarbonate removed from the body (see page 45).

Quiz 4

1 Oxygen reaches the lungs and moves down to the alveoli. It then transfers into the pulmonary capillaries and most is taken up by the haemoglobin molecules in the red cells. The oxygen is then taken to the tissues of the body where it is released. At all stages, the oxygen moves from a high to a low partial pressure (see page 47).
2 The alveolar gas is not like room air. It contains water vapour and a higher concentration of carbon dioxide. These reduce the space available for oxygen because the total pressure in the aveoli must still equal atmospheric pressure (that is, 760 mm Hg). Furthermore, oxygen is constantly leaking out of the alveoli into the surrounding capillaries (see page 47–9).
3 The factors affecting the rate of diffusion of oxygen across the

alveolar membrane are (see page 53):

- The surface area of the membrane separating the gas and blood
- The thickness of the membrane
- The difference in partial pressure of the gas across the membrane
- The size of the molecules in the gas
- The solubility of the gas in the fluid lining the alveoli
- The solubility of the gas in blood.

4 1·34 ml of oxygen per gram of haemoglobin (see page 56).

5 100 mm Hg (13·3 kPa) (see page 57).

6 There is a steep rise in SaO_2 at lower levels of PaO_2. At higher levels of PaO_2 however, the SaO_2 rises very little (see figure 4.7, page 57).

7 19·75 ml oxygen per 100 ml blood.
The oxygen content per 100 ml blood is (see page 59):

$$\text{haemoglobin concentration} \times 1{\cdot}34 \times \text{saturation} + (0{\cdot}003 \times PAO_2)$$

therefore in this case the oxygen content per 100 ml blood is:

$$15 \times 1{\cdot}34 \times 97\% + (0{\cdot}003 \times 85)$$

$$= 19{\cdot}497 \times 0{\cdot}255$$

$$= 19{\cdot}75 \text{ ml oxygen per 100 ml blood.}$$

8 Normally the PAO_2 is sufficiently high to enable most of the available spaces on the haemoglobin molecule to be filled. As a result the haemoglobin in arterial blood is almost fully saturated. Consequently any increase in oxygen content resulting from an increase in PAO_2 has to come from increasing the amount of oxygen dissolved in plasma. This amount is very small compared with the amount of oxygen associated with haemoglobin.

In contrast, if the PAO_2 is low then there will be less saturation of the haemoglobin molecule in addition to less being dissolved in plasma. The oxygen content therefore falls greatly, mainly because of the fall in the number of oxygen molecules being carried by haemoglobin.

9 790 ml oxygen per minute.
The oxygen delivery is (see page 60):

$$\text{cardiac output} \times \text{oxygen content}$$

therefore the oxygen delivery in this patient is:

$4000 \times 19{\cdot}75 = 790$ ml oxygen per minute.

10 An increase in temperature, $PaCO_2$, and hydrogen ion concentration as well as a fall in PaO_2.

Quiz 5

1 It increases (see page 65).
2 In partial compensation the body adjusts to the additional acid (or base) but does not restore the pH to normality. In these cases an acidaemia (or alkalaemia) would persist. In contrast, complete compensation means the pH has been returned to the normal range. It does not mean, however, that the underlying cause of the acid-base disturbance has gone away. In other words the acidosis (or alkalosis) remains but the acidaemia (or alkalaemia) has gone (see pages 69–70).
3 An increased acid load or an increased loss of bicarbonate (see page 76), or an impaired excretion of the normal acid lead.
4 Both decrease (see page 77).
5 Respiratory compensation and, provided the kidneys are functional, metabolic compensation (see pages 80 and 82).
6 Respiratory compensation for metabolic acidosis lowers the actual bicarbonate concentration even further. In contrast, metabolic compensation leads to increased bicarbonate retention. This partially restores the fall in standard bicarbonate concentration resulting from the metabolic acidosis but it remains below the normal range. As the standard bicarbonate increases, the actual bicarbonate will also increase.
7 Intracellular and extracellular buffers (see page 84–5).
8 This woman has an acute respiratory acidosis. She is unconscious and therefore has a strong chance of having reduced alveolar ventilation (see page 66). As a result you would expect her to be at risk of retaining carbon dioxide and developing a respiratory acidosis. Analysis of the arterial sample supports this because (see page 72):

- The pH is low, indicating that there is an acidaemia
- The $PaCO_2$ is high, indicating that there is a respiratory acidosis.
- The standard bicarbonate and base excess are slightly high.

Putting these together you can conclude that this patient has developed a respiratory acidosis secondary to her decreased consciousness. As the standard bicarbonate and base excess are increased slightly it indicates that this condition has lasted long enough to allow some renal compensation to develop. As she was previously well (that is, no history of respiratory problems) and the pH is still severely abnormal (that is, compensation is far from complete) the patient is probably suffering from an acute respiratory acidosis.

9 This woman has chronic respiratory acidosis. The history is strongly suggestive of a patient with chronic obstructive airway disease secondary to smoking (see page 73). Analysis of the arterial sample supports this because (see page 75):

- The pH is within the normal range
- The $PaCO_2$ is high, indicating there is a respiratory acidosis
- The standard bicarbonate and base excess are high.

Putting these together you can conclude that this patient has developed a respiratory acidosis. Furthermore, the raised standard bicarbonate and base excess indicates that the body has had sufficient time to develop metabolic compensation. This has brought the pH to within the normal range. Consequently, this patient demonstrates complete metabolic compensation.

10 This woman has mixed respiratory and metabolic acidosis. From the history it is likely that she has a respiratory acidosis resulting from the depressed consciousness (see page 66). In addition, the tablets she has taken can give rise to metabolic acidosis. Analysis of the arterial sample supports this because (see page 88):

- The pH is very low, indicating that there is severe acidaemia
- The $PaCO_2$ is high, indicating that there is a respiratory acidosis
- The standard bicarbonate and base excess are very low, indicating that there is a metabolic acidosis

Putting these together you can conclude that this patient has developed a mixed acidosis secondary to the dothiepin. These tablets produced a metabolic acidosis at the same time as depressing the consciousness. Initially, she may have been able to provide some respiratory compensation by blowing off extra amounts of carbon dioxide. As she began to lose consciousness, however, this ability would have been impaired and she would have begun to retain carbon dioxide. Consequently, by the time the arterial blood sample was taken, she had a combined respiratory and metabolic acidosis. For those who like using graphs you may find it interesting to plot these results on figure 5.9. You will notice she lies between the metabolic and respiratory acidosis bands.

Quiz 6

1 It falls (see page 93).
2 Respiratory alkalosis means there is an excess of base in the body because of an increase in alveolar ventilation resulting in a fall in $PACO_2$. The patient's pH may or may not be normal because there could be other factors affecting the overall hydrogen ion concentration—for example, metabolic compensation or a coexisting acidosis or alkalosis. Respiratory alkalaemia means that the excess of base in the body is sufficient to alter the patient's pH to above the normal range (see pages 93 and 94).
3 No. Normally the respiratory alkalosis is short lived so there is insufficient time to develop maximal metabolic compensation (see page 96).
4 Loss of acid (see page 99).
5 Respiratory compensation causes the actual bicarbonate concentration to rise by a small amount—that is, in the order of several mmol/l (see page 103).
6 Hypoxia. Besides increasing the $PaCO_2$, reducing alveolar ventilation will lead to a reduction in the amount of oxygen getting to the patient's circulation (see chapter 4, page 51). If this causes the PaO_2 to fall below a critical level the body will respond by stimulating respiration (see page 103).
7 Coexisting deficiencies in essential electrolytes, in particular sodium (see page 105).
8 This women is suffering from chronic respiratory alkalosis. If this high respiratory rate has been persisting for years then you would expect this patient to have developed a chronic respiratory alkalosis with metabolic compensation.

   Analysis of the arterial sample supports this because:

   - The high pH confirms there is an alkalaemia
   - The low $PaCO_2$ indicates that there is a respiratory alkalosis.
   - Both the standard bicarbonate and base excess are below normal limits.

Putting these together you can conclude that this patient has a long history of a rapid respiratory rate. Though this has produced a respiratory alkalosis it has also provided sufficient time for distinct metabolic compensation to develop. As a result the pH is just above the normal range.

9 This woman has a metabolic alkalosis. Regular aspiration of a nasogastric tube will have the same effect as vomiting—that is, there will be a net loss of gastric acid from the body. As this has been going on for 10 days a metabolic alkalosis has probably developed.

Analysis of the arterial sample supports this because:

- The high pH confirms there is an alkalaemia
- The $PaCO_2$ is high
- Both the standard bicarbonate and base excess are above normal limits.

Putting these together you can conclude that this patient has developed an alkalaemia due to a metabolic alkalosis. Her body is compensating for this by retaining carbon dioxide. As the pH remains above the normal limits, however, this respiratory compensation is only partial.

10 This man has a metabolic alkalosis. We would expect that he is likely to develop a metabolic alkalosis because of the treatment with a loop diuretic. If this is the case then respiratory compensation should have also occurred.

Analysis of the arterial sample supports this because:

- The high pH confirms there is an alkalaemia
- The high $PaCO_2$ is in keeping with respiratory compensation to a metabolic alkalosis
- The standard bicarbonate and base excess are above normal limits indicating there is a metabolic alkalosis.

Quiz 7

1 A rise in the $PaCO_2$ tends to depress the nervous system. Therefore as it rises it will lead to a fall in consciousness. In the early stages, however, you may see signs of cerebral stimulation (for example, irritability, seizures, and psychosis) as part of the group of symptoms known as hypercapnoeic encephalopathy (see page 115).

2 There is a close relationship between potassium ions and hydrogen ions in the extracellular fluid. When there is an excess

of hydrogen ions some move into the cells of the body where they are buffered by proteins and inorganic phoshates. This has the effect of slightly reducing the amount of hydrogen ions in the extracellular fluid. At the same time, however, it leads to a net increase in the positive charge moving into the cell (see figure A.1). If this was left unchecked it would increase the intracellular positive charge, damage the cell, and impair any further movement of hydrogen ions. To overcome this potassium ions move out of the cell while the hydrogen ions move in (figure A.2). This increases the potassium concentration in the extracellular fluid but it does keep the electrical charge inside the cell constant.

It follows therefore that when there are excessive amounts of hydrogen ions in the extracellular fluid there will also be high concentrations of potassium.

The exact opposite occurs when the concentration of

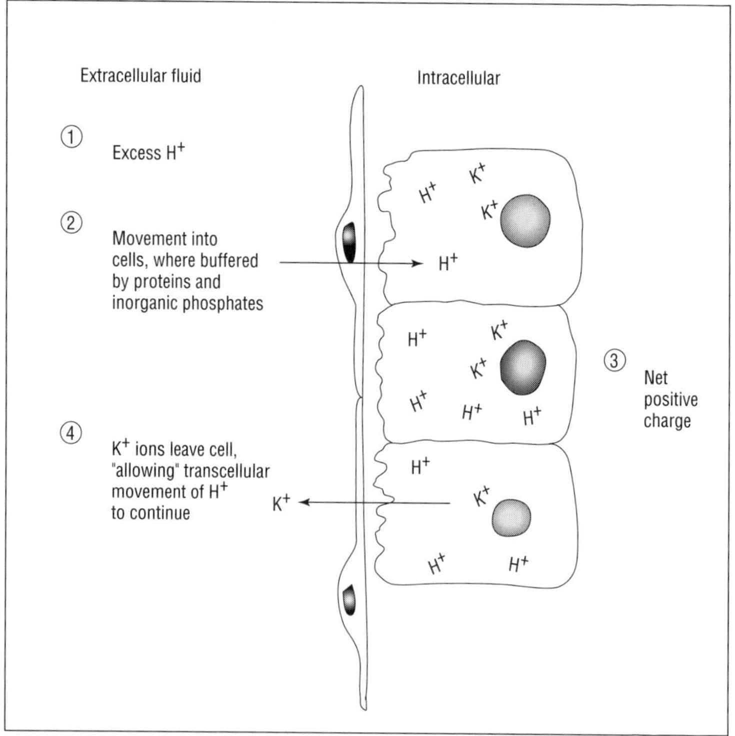

Figure A.1 Movement of H^+ to show change in intracellular charge.

hydrogen ions in the extracellular fluid is low. In these circumstances hydrogen ions move out of the cell and potassium moves in. Though this helps to move the hydrogen ion concentration nearer to the normal range it lowers the potassium concentration in the extracellular fluid (see page 100).

Consequently when there is a reduction in hydrogen ions in the extracellular fluid there will also be low concentrations of potassium.

3 This is because the mild increase of hydrogen ions results in the secretion of catecholamines. These give rise to peripheral vasoconstriction and stimulate the sweat glands in the skin.

4 Incomplete compensation is most likely because the body will not have had enough time to adapt fully to the underlying disturbance. As a result the pH will remain outside the normal range (see page 120–1).

5 The three reasons for a normal pH are (see page 121–2):

- There may not be an acid-base disturbance

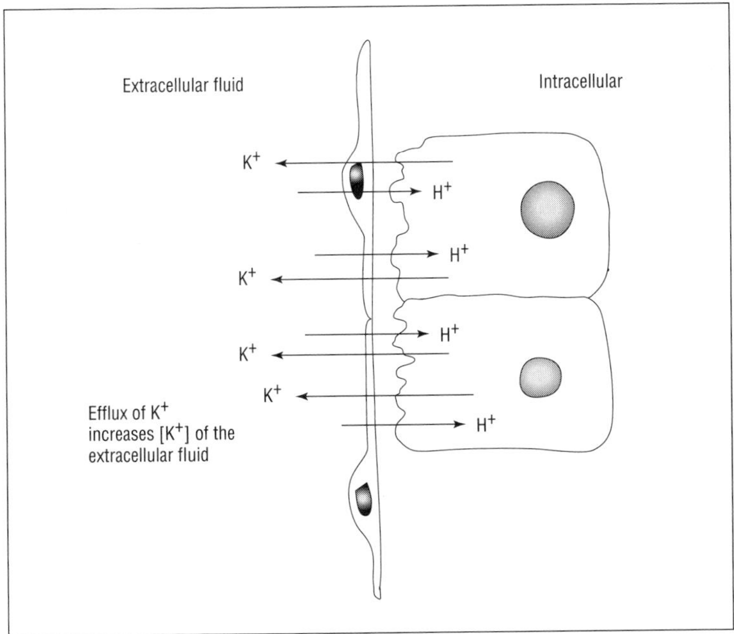

Figure A.2 Movement of H^+ and K^+ movement to indicate change in concentration in ECF.

- The body may have fully compensated for the acid-base disturbance
- There may be more than one acid-base disturbance such that they balance out one another's effect on the pH.

6 Acute or chronic respiratory acidosis

History—This patient is known to suffer from chronic obstructive pulmonary disease (COPD). This may have resulted in a chronic respiratory acidosis. She now complains of increased shortness of breath, however, presumably due to an exacerbation of her condition. Depending on how this affects her gas exchange, the respiratory acidosis may get better (if her increased respiratory rate increases the removal of CO_2) or worse (if the exacerbation impairs her ability to remove CO_2). If the respiratory acidosis improved, the $PaCO_2$ would be lower than that expected from the bicarbonate concentration. Alternatively, the $PaCO_2$ would be higher than that expected from the bicarbonate concentration if respiratory acidosis got worse. In addition, there may be elements of metabolic acidosis if her gas exchange is impaired to the point where she develops tissue hypoxia and therefore a lactic acidosis.

Systematic analysis of the blood gas results

Is there an acidaemia or alkalaemia?—As the pH is below the normal range, there is an acidaemia (see page 121).

Is there evidence of a disturbance in the respiratory component of the body's acid base balance?—Yes, the $PaCO_2$ is raised. In the light of the pH this suggests that at least a primary respiratory acidosis is present (see page 122).

Is there evidence of a disturbance in the metabolic component of the body's acid base balance?—Yes, the standard bicarbonate and base excess are raised. In the light of the pH, this is probably due to metabolic compensation for a respiratory acidosis. Alternatively, if they are reflecting a primary metabolic alkalosis then their effect on the overall pH is less than the primary respiratory acidosis (see page 126).

Is there a single or multiple acid-base disturbance?—By using the graph on page 132 we can see that the results lie on the upper edge of the chronic respiratory acidosis band.

By using the arithmetical method, if the patient had a chronic respiratory acidosis the expected actual bicarbonate would be:

$$24{\cdot}5+(0{\cdot}4\times(63{\cdot}2-40))=33{\cdot}8 \text{ mmol/l}$$

As this expected value is higher than the results obtained, then there is not just a simple chronic respiratory acidosis. If we analyse the results as if the patient has an acute respiratory acidosis, we would expect her to have an actual bicarbonate of:

$$24{\cdot}5+(0{\cdot}1\times(63{\cdot}2-40))=26{\cdot}8 \text{ mmol/l}$$

As we can see, this is much lower than the actual result, so this patient's results lie somewhere between acute and chronic respiratory acidosis.

Is the PaO_2 uptake abnormal?—By using mm Hg an inspired oxygen of 30% will have a partial pressure of:

$$30\times760/100=228 \text{ mm Hg}$$

This would mean the expected PaO_2 would be at least $228-76=152$ mm Hg.

By using kPa an inspired oxygen of 30% will have a partial pressure of about 30 kPa. This would mean the expected PaO_2 would be at least $30-10=20$ kPa. As this is higher than the actual result, there is a problem with oxygen uptake.

Integrate the clinical findings with the data interpretation

The clinical and data analysis tally. This patient could have a chronic respiratory acidosis with incomplete compensation. Alternatively, she could have a fully compensated chronic respiratory acidosis with a superimposed acute respiratory acidosis. The latter explanation is more likely, in that we know that her respiratory condition is chronic but has rapidly deteriorated over two days.

7 Metabolic acidosis and resiratory acidosis

History—This patient is suffering from an overdose and an associated epileptic fit. Dothiepin is a tricyclic antidepressant that can produce metabolic acidosis. In addition, this patient probably has a respiratory acidosis. This would be from the decreased consciousness (secondary to the medication) slowing the respiratory rate and causing poor alveolar ventilation.

Systematic analysis of the blood gas results

Is there an acidaemia or alkalaemia?—There is an acidaemia because the pH is 6·71.

Is there evidence of a disturbance in the respiratory component of the body's acid base balance?—There is a disturbance because the $PaCO_2$ is above the normal range In the light of the pH this indicates that at least part of the acidaemia is due to a respiratory acidosis.

Is there evidence of a disturbance in the metabolic component of the body's acid base balance?—Yes, the standard bicarbonate concentration is low, and the base excess concentration is very negative. In the light of the pH, this indicates that there is a metabolic acidosis and no metabolic compensation for the respiratory acidosis.

Is there a single or multiple acid-base disturbance?—By using the graph on page 132 you can see that the results lie between the metabolic and respiratory acidosis bands. This implies there is a mixed acidosis.

By using the arithmetical method, if the patient had a metabolic acidosis a 1 mmol/l fall in the actual HCO_3^- would produce a 1·0 – 1·3 mm Hg fall in $PaCO_2$. Therefore a 14 mmol/l fall in HCO_3^- would produce a 14·0 – 18·2 mm Hg fall in $PaCO_2$. Consequently if this was a simple metabolic acidosis, this patient should have a $PaCO_2$ of around 21·8 – 25·5 mm Hg (2·9 – 3·4 kPa). As the $PaCO_2$ is much higher, the arithmetical method supports the idea that there is both a respiratory acidosis and metabolic acidosis.

Is the PaO_2 uptake abnormal?—There is evidence of a defect when we calculate the expected PaO_2 in a patient breathing 85% oxygen. By using mm Hg an inspired oxygen of 85% will have a partial pressure of $85 \times 760/100 = 646$ mm Hg. This would mean the expected PaO_2 would be at least $646 - 76 = 570$ mm Hg. By using kPa an inspired oxygen of 85% will have a partial pressure of about 85 kPa. This would mean the expected PaO_2 would be at least $85 - 10 = 75$ kPa.

As we can see, the patient's results do not tally with this, therefore there is a defect in oxygen uptake.

Integrate the clinical findings with the data interpretation

The clinical suspicion and the data analysis agree. This patient has a combined acidosis. The inadequate alveolar ventilation is giving rise to the respiratory acidosis as well as to hypoxaemia. The lack of oxygen in the blood stream leads to hypoxia and anaerobic metabolism. As a result metabolic acidosis develops because there is a rise in the production of lactic acid. In addition, both the fit and the tricyclic medication will independently produce a metabolic acidosis.

8 Metabolic acidosis and respiratory alkalosis.

History—This patient is known to have insulin dependent diabetes. Any physiological insult—for example, infection or surgery—can affect the control of the patient's blood sugar. This patient probably has a chest infection, and we might expect this to result in a metabolic acidosis as a result of loss of diabetic control. This should provoke respiratory compensation, with a decrease in $PaCO_2$.

The chest infection itself, however, may produce an independent disturbance in the patient's acid-base status. The infection can stimulate the pulmonary receptors and lead to an increase in respiratory rates (see page 95). Furthermore, if the infection is severe enough to make the patient hypoxic, then this will also stimulate an increase in respiration. In either case, the patient will eliminate additional carbon dioxide and produce a respiratory alkalosis. A further acid-base disturbance could occur in this patient if he had hypoxia severe enough to produce lactic acidosis.

Systematic analysis of the blood gas results

Is there an acidaemia or alkalaemia—As the pH is just within normal limits, there is no acidaemia or alkalaemia.

Is there evidence of a disturbance in the respiratory component of the body's acid base balance?—There is a disturbance because the $PaCO_2$ is lowered. In the light of the pH, this could indicate either a primary respiratory alkalosis that has been fully compensated for or a primary metabolic acidosis that has been fully compensated for. Alternatively, there could be both a primary respiratory alkalosis and a primary metabolic acidosis that are having equal but opposite effects on the pH.

Is there evidence of a disturbance in the metabolic component of the body's acid base balance?—Yes, because both the standard bicarbonate and base excess concentrations are lowered. In the light of the pH, this indicates that any of the above explanations could be present.

Is there a single or multiple acid-base disturbance?—By using the graph on page 132 you can see that the results lie at the junction of chronic respiratory alkalosis and metabolic acidosis.

By using the arithmetical method, if the patient had a chronic respiratory alkalosis the expected actual bicarbonate would be:

$$24{\cdot}5 - (0{\cdot}5 \times (40 - 22{\cdot}7)) = 15{\cdot}9 \text{ mmol/l}$$

As this expected value is higher than the results obtained, then there is not just a simple chronic respiratory alkalosis.

If we analyse the results as if the patient has a metabolic acidosis, we would expect him to have a $PaCO_2$ between:

$$(40 - (1{\cdot}3 \times (24{\cdot}5 - 15{\cdot}1))) \quad \text{and} \quad (40 - (1{\cdot}0 \times (24{\cdot}5 - 15{\cdot}1))) \text{ mm Hg}$$

that is,

$$27{\cdot}8 - 30{\cdot}6 \text{ mm mmHg } (3{\cdot}7 - 4{\cdot}0 \text{ kPa})$$

Again this does not tally with the patient's result, adding further support to the idea that more than one acid-base disturbance is present.

Is the PaO_2 uptake abnormal?—A patient breathing room air should have PaO_2 of more than 90 mm Hg (12 kPa). As this patient is also hyperventilating, we would expect his PaO_2 to be at the upper range of normal. As the patient's result is below the lower range of normal there is a problem with oxygen uptake.

Integrate the clinical findings with the data interpretation

The clinical and data analysis tally. The patient has a chest infection, which has caused his diabetes to become uncontrolled, leading to a metabolic acidosis.

In addition, respiration is being stimulated even more because of the action of the chest infection on the pulmonary receptors. Further stimulation due to the low oxygen uptake may also be present, but this is unlikely. The resulting increase in his minute volume will give rise to a primary respiratory alkalosis. As a result of the primary respiratory alkalosis, his $PaCO_2$ is at a lower value than would have been produced by simple respiratory compensation for a metabolic acidosis.

This patient therefore has three acid-base disturbances: a primary respiratory alkalosis, a primary metabolic acidosis, and respiratory compensation for the metabolic acidosis. The end result of this combination is that the patient's pH lies within normal limits.

9 Combined respiratory alkalosis and metabolic acidosis with slight impairment in oxygen uptake.

History

This patient probably developed a combined respiratory and metabolic acidosis during the time of the cardiac arrest. After the successful resuscitation, however, the additional carbon dioxide would have been removed and she may simply be left with a metabolic acidosis. Patients who have a cardiac arrest are at risk of aspirating. Consequently she may have evidence of impaired oxygen uptake. Furthermore, there could be other acid-base abnormalities present depending on her state of health before the arrest.

Systematic analysis of the blood gas results

Is there an acidaemia or alkalaemia? As the pH is just within the normal range, there is neither an acidaemia nor an alkalaemia.

Is there evidence of a disturbance in the respiratory component of the body's acid base balance?—Yes, the $PaCO_2$ is low. In the light of the pH, this could mean that there is a primary respiratory alkalosis with full metabolic compensation. Alternatively, a primary metabolic acidosis may be present with full respiratory compensation.

Is there evidence of a disturbance in the metabolic component of the body's acid base balance?—Yes, the standard bicarbonate and base excess are low. This is in keeping with either of the possibilities mentioned above.

Is there a single or multiple acid-base disturbance?—By using the graph on page 132 you can see that the results lie between the normal bands associated with a chronic respiratory alkalosis.

By using the arithmetical method, if the patient had a chronic respiratory alkalosis the expected actual HCO_3 would be:

$$(24{\cdot}5 + (0{\cdot}5 \times (40 - 15{\cdot}9))) = 12{\cdot}45 \text{ mmol/l}$$

This is just above the value obtained from the patient and therefore supports the diagnosis of a chronic respiratory alkalosis. There are no indicators in the history, however, that this patient has such a condition. It is therefore more likely that she has a mixed respiratory alkalosis and metabolic acidosis with a resultant pH that lies coincidentally in a band associated with chronic respiratory alkalosis.

Is the PaO_2 uptake abnormal?—There is evidence of a slight defect when we calculate the expected PaO_2 in a patient breathing 100% oxygen. By using mm Hg an inspired oxygen of 100% will have a partial pressure of $100 \times 760/100 = 760$ mm Hg. This would mean the expected PaO_2 would be at least $760 - 76 = 684$ mm Hg. By using kPa an inspired oxygen of 100% will have a partial pressure of about 100 kPa. This would mean the expected PaO_2 would be at least $100 - 10 = 90$ kPa.

As the patient's results are slightly lower than predicted, there is a problem with oxygen uptake.

Integrate the clinical findings with the data interpretation

The clinical and data analysis tally. This patient has a metabolic acidosis after the cardiac arrest. The mechanical ventilation is greater than that required to remove the carbon dioxide generated by metabolism. As a result the patient has developed a primary respiratory alkalosis as well. There is evidence of a slight impairment of oxygen uptake, but this would be insufficient to cause inadequate tissue hypoxia.

10 Combined respiratory and metabolic alkalosis with iadequate oxygen uptake.

History

This patient has probably developed a metabolic alkalosis because of the loss of gastric acid in the nasogastric aspirate. Provided this is the only acid-base disturbance and she has been receiving adequate intravenous fluids, then we would expect respiratory compensation to have developed. If she is hypovolaemic, however, then she may have a metabolic acidosis as well because of the production of lactic acid from the ischaemic tissues.

We know that oxygen uptake decreases with age. This could be further compromised by any pulmonary pathology that may have been pre-existing or occurred after the operation (for example, aspiration). In these circumstances there could be a coexisting respiratory acidosis (due to carbon dioxide retention) or respiratory alkalosis (due to additional carbon dioxide removal).

Systematic analysis of the blood gas results

Is there an acidaemia or alkalaemia?—The pH is above the normal range, indicating there is an alkalaemia.

Is there evidence of a disturbance in the respiratory component of the body's acid-base balance?—The $PaCO_2$ is within normal limits. In the light of the pH, this could mean that there is a metabolic alkalosis that is uncompensated. As there has been sufficient time for compensation to develop there is probably a coexisting respiratory alkalosis that is preventing appropriate respiratory compensation.

Is there evidence of a disturbance in the metabolic component of the body's acid-base balance?—Yes the standard bicarbonate and base excess are raised. In the light of the pH and $PaCO_2$, this means that a primary metabolic alkalosis exists.

Is there a single or multiple acid-base disturbance?—By using the graph on page 132 you can see that the results lie just outside the standard band associated with metabolic alkalosis. By using the arithmetical method, if the patient had simply a metabolic alkalosis the expected $PaCO_2$ would be

$$40 + (0{\cdot}6 \times (34{\cdot}5 - 24{\cdot}5)) = 45{\cdot}7 \text{ mm Hg } (6{\cdot}0 \text{ kPa})$$

This is a lot higher than that found in the patient, indicating that additional carbon dioxide is being removed. Consequently, there is probably a coexisting respiratory alkalosis.

Is the PaO_2 uptake abnormal?—There is evidence of a defect when we calculate the expected PaO_2 in a patient breathing 45% oxygen. By using mm Hg an inspired oxygen of 45% will have a partial pressure of $45 \times 760/100 = 342$ mm Hg. This would mean the expected PaO_2 would be at least $342 - 76 = 266$ mm Hg. By using kPa an inspired oxygen of 45% would have a partial pressure of approximately 45 kPa. This would mean the expected PaO_2 would be at least $45 - 10 = 35$ kPa.

As these calculated levels are considerably lower than those found in the patient, there is a problem with oxygen uptake.

Integrate the clinical findings with the data interpretation

The clinical and data analysis tally. The expected metabolic alkalosis is present but there is a coexisting respiratory alkalosis as well. This is probably due to stimulation of the pulmonary receptors leading to hyperventilation. Support for this patient having coexisting pulmonary pathology comes from the low PaO_2 result in the light of the inspired oxygen concentration.

Self assessment quiz

TERRY BROWN, PETER DRISCOLL

What acid-base abnormalities are present in the following cases (answers on page 179)?

Question 1

A 65 year old man with COAD presented to the emergency department with a 48 hour history of worsening dyspnoea. While he was breathing room air, an arterial sample was taken for blood gas analysis. The results were:

Measure	Normal range	Result
pH	7·36–7·44	7·32
$PaCO_2$	35–45 mm Hg (4·7–6·0 kPa)	55·7 mm Hg (7·4 kPa)
Actual HCO_3^-	21–28 mmol/l	28·3 mmol/l
Standard HCO_3^-	21–27 mmol/l	26·2 mmol/l
Base excess	±2 mmol/l	1·0 mmol/l
PaO_2	Over 90 mm Hg (12·0 kPa) on room air	67·9 mm Hg (9·1 kPa)

Question 2

A 75 year old woman who was known to have bronchial carcinoma presented to the emergency department with increasing drowsiness. While she was breathing 25% oxygen via a mask, an arterial sample was taken for blood gas analysis. The results were:

Measure	Normal range	Result
pH	7·36–7·44	7·33
$PaCO_2$	35–45 mm Hg (4·7–6·0 kPa)	70·4 mm Hg (9·3 kPa)
Actual HCO_3^-	21–28 mmol/l	36·6 mmol/l
Standard HCO_3^-	21–27 mmol/l	32·5 mmol/l
Base excess	±2 mmol/l	7·4 mmol/l
PaO_2	Over 90 mm Hg (12·0 kPa) on room air	33·0 mm Hg (4·4 kPa)

Question 3

A 17 year old woman was brought to the emergency department after falling from a horse and suffering a head injury. When she was in the department she became increasingly drowsy. While she was breathing 80% oxygen via a non-rebreathing mask with reservoir, an arterial sample was taken for blood gas analysis. The results were:

Measure	Normal range	Result
pH	7·36–7·44	7·17
$PaCO_2$	35–45 mm Hg (4·7–6·0 kPa)	80·4 mm Hg (10·6 kPa)
Actual HCO_3^-	21–28 mmol/l	28·5 mmol/l
Standard HCO_3^-	21–27 mmol/l	23·9 mmol/l
Base excess	±2 mmol/l	−2·5 mmol/l
PaO_2	Over 90 mm Hg (12·0 kPa) on room air	119·9 mm Hg (15·8 kPa)

Question 4

A 24 year old man who was known to suffer from epilepsy was brought to the emergency department in status epilepticus. This was treated successfully with intravenous diazepam. Immediately afterwards while he was breathing room air, an arterial sample was taken for blood gas analysis. The results were:

Measure	Normal range	Result
pH	7·36–7·44	6·99
$PaCO_2$	35–45 mm Hg (4·7–6·0 kPa)	26·8 mm Hg (3·5 kPa)
Actual HCO_3^-	21–28 mmol/l	6·1 mmol/l
Standard HCO_3^-	21–27 mmol/l	6·0 mmol/l
Base excess	±2 mmol/l	−23·6 mmol/l
PaO_2	Over 90 mm Hg (12·0 kPa) on room air	165·3 mm Hg (21·8 kPa)

Question 5

A 46 year old man who was known to be diabetic was brought to the emergency department complaining of feeling generally unwell, with fever and vomiting. His blood sugar was 38·0 mmol/l; his urea and electrolytes were within the normal range. While he was breathing 40% oxygen via a mask, an arterial sample was taken for blood gas analysis. The results were:

Measure	Normal range	Result
pH	7·36–7·44	7·02
$PaCO_2$	35–45 mm Hg (4·7–6·0 kPa)	22 mm Hg (2·9 kPa)
Actual HCO_3^-	21–28 mmol/l	6·1 mmol/l
Standard HCO_3^-	21–27 mmol/l	6·0 mmol/l
Base excess	±2 mmol/l	−23 mmol/l
PaO_2	Over 90 mm Hg (12·0 kPa) on room air	274 mm Hg (36 kPa)

Question 6

A 60 year old woman was brought to the emergency department complaining of chest pain. Shortly after arrival she suffered a cardiac arrest. After 5 minutes of resuscitation she developed return of spontaneous circulation and began to breathe spontaneously. While she was breathing 85% oxygen via a bag-valve-mask system, an arterial sample was taken for blood gas analysis. The results were:

Measure	Normal range	Result
pH	7·36–7·44	7·11
$PaCO_2$	35–45 mm Hg (4·7–6·0 kPa)	21·6 mm Hg (2·8 kPa)
Actual HCO_3^-	21–28 mmol/l	7·0 mmol/l
Standard HCO_3^-	21–27 mmol/l	6·5 mmol/l
Base excess	±2 mmol/l	−21·8 mmol/l
PaO_2	Over 90 mm Hg (12·0 kPa) on room air	507·9 mm Hg (66·8 kPa)

Question 7

An 85 year old woman presented to the emergency department with a four day history of feeling generally unwell with fever, cough, and shortness of breath. While she was breathing 30% oxygen via a mask, an arterial sample was taken for blood gas analysis. The results were:

Measure	Normal range	Result
pH	7·36–7·44	7·22
$PaCO_2$	35–45 mm Hg (4·7–6·0 kPa)	18·2 mm Hg (2·4 kPa)
Actual HCO_3^-	21–28 mmol/l	7·7 mmol/l
Standard HCO_3^-	21–27 mmol/l	7·0 mmol/l
Base excess	±2 mmol/l	−19·1 mmol/l
PaO_2	Over 90 mm Hg (12·0 kPa) on room air	115·6 mm Hg (15 kPa)

Question 8

A 74 year old man presented to the emergency department with a three day history of feeling generally unwell with fever and rigors. While he was breathing room air, an arterial sample was taken for blood gas analysis. The results were:

Measure	Normal range	Result
pH	7·36–7·44	7·30
$PaCO_2$	35–45 mm Hg (4·7–6·0 kPa)	24·3 mm Hg (3·2 kPa)
Actual HCO_3^-	21–28 mmol/l	12·2 mmol/l
Standard HCO_3^-	21–27 mmol/l	14·5 mmol/l
Base excess	±2 mmol/l	−12·9 mmol/l
PaO_2	Over 90 mm Hg (12·0 kPa) on room air	99·3 mm Hg (13 kPa)

Question 9

A 24 year old man who was known to be an alcohol misuser presented to the emergency department with a 24 hour history of severe abdominal pain. On examination, he was tender in the epigastrium. His urea and electrolytes were normal, but his amylase was 2400 IU/l. While he was breathing room air, an arterial sample was taken for blood gas analysis. The results were:

Measure	Normal range	Result
pH	7·36–7·44	7·31
$PaCO_2$	35–45 mm Hg (4·7–6·0 kPa)	25·2 mm Hg (3·3 kPa)
Actual HCO_3^-	21–28 mmol/l	8·7 mmol/l
Standard HCO_3^-	21–27 mmol/l	8·0 mmol/l
Base excess	±2 mmol/l	−19·3 mmol/l
PaO_2	Over 90 mm Hg (12·0 kPa) on room air	114·4 mm Hg (15 kPa)

Question 10

A 70 year old woman was brought to the emergency department after having collapsed at home. She was witnessed to have a grand mal seizure after the collapse which had lasted for 10 minutes. On examination she was drowsy and febrile. Urea, electrolytes, and blood sugar were all in the normal range. She had a raised white cell count. While she was breathing 60% oxygen via a mask, an arterial sample was taken for blood gas analysis. The results were:

Measure	Normal range	Result
pH	7·36–7·44	7·08
$PaCO_2$	35–45 mm Hg (4·7–6·0 kPa)	21·2 mm Hg (2·8 kPa)
Actual HCO_3^-	21–28 mmol/l	6·7 mmol/l
Standard HCO_3^-	21–27 mmol/l	6·0 mmol/l
Base excess	±2 mmol/l	−22·0 mmol/l
PaO_2	Over 90 mm Hg (12·0 kPa) on room air	351·2 mm Hg (42 kPa)

Question 11

A 44 year old man attended the emergency department complaining of pleuritic chest pain and dyspnoea for the previous two days. On examination he was breathless at rest and had a large pneumothorax. While he was breathing 60% oxygen via a mask, an arterial sample was taken for blood gas analysis. The results were:

Measure	Normal range	Result
pH	7·36–7·44	7·44
$PaCO_2$	35–45 mm Hg (4·7–6·0 kPa)	27·1 mm Hg (3·6 kPa)
Actual HCO_3^-	21–28 mmol/l	17·9 mmol/l
Standard HCO_3^-	21–27 mmol/l	20·5 mmol/l
Base excess	±2 mmol/l	−4·6 mmol/l
PaO_2	Over 90 mm Hg (12·0 kPa) on room air	92·5 mm Hg (12·2 kPa)

Question 12

A 32 year old woman attended the emergency department complaining of shortness of breath and some pleuritic chest pain for the previous 48 hours. She had recently had an operation on her Achilles tendon and was in a below knee plaster of Paris cast. While she was breathing 60% oxygen via a mask, an arterial sample was taken for blood gas analysis. The results were:

Measure	Normal range	Result
pH	7·36–7·44	7·48
$PaCO_2$	35–45 mm Hg (4·7–6·0 kPa)	25·8 mm Hg (3·4 kPa)
Actual HCO_3^-	21–28 mmol/l	18·9 mmol/l
Standard HCO_3^-	21–27 mmol/l	21·5 mmol/l
Base excess	±2 mmol/l	−2·8 mmol/l
PaO_2	Over 90 mm Hg (12·0 kPa) on room air	106·8 mm Hg (14·0 kPa)

Question 13

A 39 year old man who was known to suffer from chronic pancreatitis presented to the emergency department complaining of severe abdominal pain for the previous two days. On examination he was agitated and in severe pain. His urea and electrolytes were within normal limits. While he was breathing room air, an arterial sample was taken for blood gas analysis. The results were:

Measure	Normal range	Result
pH	7·36–7·44	7·43
$PaCO_2$	35–45 mm Hg (4·7–6·0 kPa)	20·9 mm Hg (2·8 kPa)
Actual HCO_3^-	21–28 mmol/l	14·5 mmol/l
Standard HCO_3^-	21–27 mmol/l	17·2 mmol/l
Base excess	±2 mmol/l	−8·4 mmol/l
PaO_2	Over 90 mm Hg (12·0 kPa) on room air	110·5 mm Hg (14·5 kPa)

Question 14

A 15 year old youth with asthma attended the emergency department complaining of an acute exacerbation of his asthma. On examination, he was distressed, tachypnoeic, and wheezy. While he was breathing 40% oxygen via a mask, an arterial sample was taken for blood gas analysis. The results were:

Measure	Normal range	Result
pH	7·36–7·44	7·59
$PaCO_2$	35–45 mm Hg (4·7–6·0 kPa)	22·6 mm Hg (3·0 kPa)
Actual HCO_3^-	21–28 mmol/l	21·1 mmol/l
Standard HCO_3^-	21–27 mmol/l	23·5 mmol/l
Base excess	±2 mmol/l	1·4 mmol/l
PaO_2	Over 90 mm Hg (12·0 kPa) on room air	162·1 mm Hg (21·3 kPa)

Question 15

A 58 year old man was brought to the emergency department after taking an overdose of dothiepin tablets. On examination he was conscious and agitated. He was cardiovascularly stable. While he was breathing room air, an arterial sample was taken for blood gas analysis. The results were:

Measure	Normal range	Result
pH	7·36–7·44	7·58
$PaCO_2$	35–45 mm Hg (4·7–6·0 kPa)	21·5 mm Hg (2·8 kPa)
Actual HCO_3^-	21–28 mmol/l	20·1 mmol/l
Standard HCO_3^-	21–27 mmol/l	23·2 mmol/l
Base excess	±2 mmol/l	0·6 mmol/l
PaO_2	Over 90 mm Hg (12·0 kPa) on room air	95 mm Hg (12·5 kPa)

Question 16

A 37 year old woman who was known to be asthmatic presented to the emergency department complaining of an acute exacerbation of her asthma. On examination she was breathless at rest, with poor air entry and widespread wheeze. While she was breathing 60% oxygen via a mask, an arterial sample was taken for blood gas analysis. The results were:

Measure	Normal range	Result
pH	7·36–7·44	7·71
$PaCO_2$	35–45 mm Hg (4·7–6·0 kPa)	12·2 mm Hg (1·6 kPa)
Actual HCO_3^-	21–28 mmol/l	15·1 mmol/l
Standard HCO_3^-	21–27 mmol/l	21·7 mmol/l
Base excess	±2 mmol/l	−4·5 mmol/l
PaO_2	Over 90 mm Hg (12·0 kPa) on room air	161·8 mm Hg (21·3 kPa)

Question 17

A 44 year old woman who was known to be asthmatic was brought to the emergency department with an acute exacerbation of her asthma. On examination whe was unable to speak and appeared obtunded. While she was breathing 80% oxygen via a non-rebreathing mask with reservoir, an arterial sample was taken for blood gas analysis. The results were:

Measure	Normal range	Result
pH	7·36–7·44	6·82
$PaCO_2$	35–45 mm Hg (4·7–6·0 kPa)	116·8 mm Hg (15·3 kPa)
Actual HCO_3^-	21–28 mmol/l	17·6 mmol/l
Standard HCO_3^-	21–27 mmol/l	17·0 mmol/l
Base excess	±2 mmol/l	−19·6 mmol/l
PaO_2	Over 90 mm Hg (12·0 kPa) on room air	228·8 mm Hg (30 kPa)

Question 18

A 60 year old woman was brought to the emergency department at 4 am complaining of acute shortness of breath. She was known to have ischaemic heart disease. On examination she was tachypnoeic, with fine inspiratory crepitations to her mid-zones. While she was breathing 60% oxygen via a mask, an arterial sample was taken for blood gas analysis. The results were:

Measure	Normal range	Result
pH	7·36–7·44	6.98
$PaCO_2$	35–45 mm Hg (4·7–6·0 kPa)	78·7 mm Hg (10·4 kPa)
Actual HCO_3^-	21–28 mmol/l	18·8 mmol/l
Standard HCO_3^-	21–27 mmol/l	14·2 mmol/l
Base excess	±2 mmol/l	−14·7 mmol/l
PaO_2	Over 90 mm Hg (12·0 kPa) on room air	72·8 mm Hg (9·6 kPa)

Question 19

A 70 year old man was brought to the emergency department complaining of acute shortness of breath and cough. He was known to suffer from ischaemic heart disease. On examination he was clammy and cold, with fine inspiratory crepitations at both lung bases. While he was breathing 80% oxygen via a non-rebreathing mask with reservoir, an arterial sample was taken for blood gas analysis. The results were:

Measure	Normal range	Result
pH	7·36–7·44	7·09
$PaCO_2$	35–45 mm Hg (4·7–6·0 kPa)	72·1 mm Hg (9·5 kPa)
Actual HCO_3^-	21–28 mmol/l	21·3 mmol/l
Standard HCO_3^-	21–27 mmol/l	16·3 mmol/l
Base excess	±2 mmol/l	−10 mmol/l
PaO_2	Over 90 mm Hg (12·0 kPa) on room air	58·8 mm Hg (7·7 kPa)

Question 20

An 87 year old man presented to the emergency department complaining of several days' history of cough, fever, and shortness of breath. He was known to have hypertension and was receiving diuretic therapy. Blood was sent for urea and electrolytes and revealed: Na 125 mmol/l, K 3·3 mmol/l. While he was breathing room air, an arterial sample was taken for blood gas analysis. The results were:

Measure	Normal range	Result
pH	7·36–7·44	7·54
$PaCO_2$	35–45 mm Hg (4·7–6·0 kPa)	33·9 mm Hg (4·5 kPa)
Actual HCO_3^-	21–28 mmol/l	29·2 mmol/l
Standard HCO_3^-	21–27 mmol/l	30·1 mmol/l
Base excess	±2 mmol/l	6·6 mmol/l
PaO_2	Over 90 mm Hg (12·0 kPa) on room air	49·2 mm Hg (6·5 kPa)

Question 21

A 29 year old woman who was known to have insulin dependent diabetes mellitus (IDDM) presented to the emergency department complaining of a 36 hour history of shortness of breath, pleuritic chest pain, and feeling generally unwell. She took the contraceptive pill and her insulin but was on no other medications. On examination she was distressed and tachypnoeic, and her glucose monitoring stick read "over" 20 mmol/l. While she was breathing 40% oxygen via a mask, an arterial sample was taken for blood gas analysis. The results were:

Measure	Normal range	Result
pH	7·36–7·44	7·39
$PaCO_2$	35–45 mm Hg (4·7–6·0 kPa)	27·0 mm Hg (3·6 kPa)
Actual HCO_3^-	21–28 mmol/l	16·6 mmol/l
Standard HCO_3^-	21–27 mmol/l	18·6 mmol/l
Base excess	±2 mmol/l	−7·6 mmol/l
PaO_2	Over 90 mm Hg (12·0 kPa) on room air	97·4 mm Hg (12·9 kPa)

Question 22

A 19 year old man who was known to misuse drugs was brought to the emergency department after he was found unconscious at home. He had vomited and aspirated, and when the paramedic team reached him he had suffered a cardiorespiratory arrest. He had responded to resuscitation, and on arrival in the department had return of spontaneous circulation, but he was still being ventilated via an endotracheal tube. While he was breathing 100% oxygen via a bag-valve-mask system, an arterial sample was taken for blood gas analysis. The results were:

Measure	Normal range	Result
pH	7·36–7·44	7·40
$PaCO_2$	35–45 mm Hg (4·7–6·0 kPa)	26·8 mm Hg (3·5 kPa)
Actual HCO_3^-	21–28 mmol/l	16·7 mmol/l
Standard HCO_3^-	21–27 mmol/l	18·6 mmol/l
Base excess	±2 mmol/l	−6·8 mmol/l
PaO_2	Over 90 mm Hg (12·0 kPa) on room air	538·8 mm Hg (70·9 kPa)

Question 23

A 65 year old man who was known to suffer from epilepsy was brought to the department by ambulance because of frequent seizures that morning. On arrival in the emergency department he had a further fit, which resolved spontaneously. His relatives said that he had had a cough and a high temperature for the previous 48 hours. On examination he was postictal, with poor air entry at both bases. While he was breathing 40% oxygen via a mask, an arterial sample was taken for blood gas analysis. The results were:

Measure	Normal range	Result
pH	7·36–7·44	7·37
$PaCO_2$	35–45 mm Hg (4·7–6·0 kPa)	28·5 mm Hg (3·8 kPa)
Actual HCO_3^-	21–28 mmol/l	17·2 mmol/l
Standard HCO_3^-	21–27 mmol/l	17·9 mmol/l
Base excess	±2 mmol/l	−7·2 mmol/l
PaO_2	Over 90 mm Hg (12·0 kPa) on room air	109·6 mm Hg (14·5 kPa)

Question 24

A 78 year old woman who was known to suffer from COAD presented to the emergency department complaining of a 48 hour history of worsening dyspnoea and cough. On examination she had decreased air entry in all areas, with widespread expiratory wheeze. Her urea and electrolytes were normal. While she was breathing room air, an arterial sample was taken for blood gas analysis. The results were:

Measure	Normal range	Result
pH	7·36–7·44	7·37
$PaCO_2$	35–45 mm Hg (4·7–6·0 kPa)	63·1 mm Hg (8·3 kPa)
Actual HCO_3^-	21–28 mmol/l	36·0 mmol/l
Standard HCO_3^-	21–27 mmol/l	32·4 mmol/l
Base excess	±2 mmol/l	8·1 mmol/l
PaO_2	Over 90 mm Hg (12·0 kPa) on room air	80·0 mm Hg (10·5 kPa)

Question 25

A 65 year old man who was known to suffer from COAD presented to the emergency department complaining of increasing shortness of breath and fever. On examination he was febrile and had decreased air entry at the left base. Electrolytes were normal. While he was breathing room air, an arterial sample was taken for blood gas analysis. The results were:

Measure	Normal range	Result
pH	7·36–7·44	7·44
$PaCO_2$	35–45 mm Hg (4·7–6·0 kPa)	54·7 mm Hg (7·2 kPa)
Actual HCO_3^-	21–28 mmol/l	36 mmol/l
Standard HCO_3^-	21–27 mmol/l	32 mmol/l
Base excess	±2 mmol/l	9·7 mmol/l
PaO_2	Over 90 mm Hg (12·0 kPa) on room air	67·0 mm Hg (8·8 kPa)

Question 26

A 42 year old man was brought to the department after taking an overdose of tricyclic antidepressants. Shortly after arrival he had protracted grand mal convulsions, which responded to repeat doses of diazepam. While he was breathing 80% oxygen via a non-rebreathing mask with reservoir, an arterial sample was taken for blood gas analysis. The results were:

Measure	Normal range	Result
pH	7·36–7·44	6·97
$PaCO_2$	35–45 mm Hg (4·7–6·0 kPa)	46·3 mm Hg (6·1 kPa)
Actual HCO_3^-	21–28 mmol/l	10·1 mmol/l
Standard HCO_3^-	21–27 mmol/l	6·4 mmol/l
Base excess	±2 mmol/l	−21·5 mmol/l
PaO_2	Over 90 mm Hg (12·0 kPa) on room air	152·8 mm Hg (20 kPa)

He was then intubated and ventilated and given 50 ml of 8·4% $NaHCO_3$. Twenty minutes later, while he was breathing 100% oxygen, an arterial sample was taken for blood gas analysis. The results were:

Measure	Normal range	Result
pH	7·36–7·44	7·45
$PaCO_2$	35–45 mm Hg (4·7–6·0 kPa)	25·3 mm Hg (3·3 kPa)
Actual HCO_3^-	21–28 mmol/l	17·7 mmol/l
Standard HCO_3^-	21–27 mmol/l	7·2 mmol/l
Base excess	±2 mmol/l	−17 mmol/l
PaO_2	Over 90 mm Hg (12·0 kPa) on room air	366·1 mm Hg (48·2 kPa)

Answers to the self assessment quiz

Question 1

Chronic respiratory acidosis. By using the graph, the results lie within the band for chronic respiratory acidosis plus hypoxia. By using the arithmetic model, we would expect an HCO_3 of 26·0 mmol/l if the acidosis was acute and 30·8 mmol/l if the acidosis was fully compensated. Hence, this patient lies between the two—that is, he is only partially compensating for the acidosis, a fact that is reflected by the pH. The PaO_2 is less than normal for a patient breathing room air.

Question 2

Chronic respiratory acidosis plus hypoxia. By using the graph, the results lie within the band for chronic respiratory acidosis. By using the arithmetic model, we would expect an HCO_3 of 36·66 mmol/l, which is exactly what the actual values are. The PaO_2 should be at least 114 mm Hg (15 kPa).

Question 3

Acute respiratory acidosis plus hypoxia. By using the graph, the results lie within this band. By using the arithmetic model, we would expect the HCO_3 to be 28·5 mmol/l, which is the same as the actual results. The PaO_2 should be at least 570 mm Hg (75 kPa).

Question 4

Metabolic acidosis and mild respiratory acidosis. By using the graph, the results lie at the edge of the band for metabolic acidosis.

By using the arithmetic model we would expect the $PaCO_2$ to be 16·1 – 21·6 mmHg (2·1 – 2·9 kPa). As it is slightly higher than this we can see that the patient has a degree of respiratory acidosis, presumably as a result of respiratory muscle fatigue and hypoxia.

Question 5

Metabolic acidosis. By using the graph, the results lie within this band. By using the arithmetic model, we would expect a $PaCO_2$ of 16·1–21·6 mm Hg (2·1 – 2·8 kPa). As we can see, the actual results match those expected for a metabolic acidosis with early partial compensation.

Question 6

Metabolic acidosis. By using the graph, the results lie within this band. By using the arithmetic model, we would expect a $PaCO_2$ of 17·3–22·5 mm Hg (2·3–2·9 kPa). As we can see, the actual results match those expected for a metabolic acidosis with early partial compensation.

Question 7

Metabolic acidosis plus hypoxia. By using the graph, the results lie within this band. By using the arithmetic model we would expect a $PaCO_2$ of 18·2–23·2 mm Hg (2·4–3·0 kPa). As we can see, the actual results match those expected for a metabolic acidosis with full compensation. The expected PaO_2 is 152 mm Hg (20 kPa).

Question 8

Metabolic acidosis. By using the graph, the results lie within this band. By using the arithmetic model, we would expect a $PaCO_2$ of 24·0–27·7 mm Hg (3·2–3·6 kPa). As we can see, the actual results match those expected for a metabolic acidosis with full compensation.

Question 9

Metabolic acidosis. By using the graph, the results lie within this band. By using the arithmetic model, we would expect a $PaCO_2$ of 19·5–24·2 mm Hg (2·3–3·2 kPa). As we can see, the actual results match those expected for a metabolic acidosis with minimal compensation.

Question 10

Metabolic acidosis. By using the graph, the results lie within this band. By using the arithmetic model, we would expect a $PaCO_2$ of 16·9–22·2 mm Hg (2·2–2·9 kPa). As we can see, the actual results match those expected for a metabolic acidosis with minimal early compensation.

Question 11

Chronic respiratory alkalosis plus hypoxia. By using the graph, the results lie within this band. By using the arithmetic model, we would expect the patient's actual HCO_3 to be 18·0 mmol/l. As we can see, the results match this. The patient's PaO_2 should be at least 380 mm Hg (50 kPa).

Question 12

Chronic respiratory alkalosis plus hypoxia. By using the graph, the results lie within this band. By using the arithmetic model, we would expect the patient's actual HCO_3 to be 17·4 mmol/l if fully compensated and 22·1 mmol/l if acute. As we can see, the results match those expected for a partially compensated respiratory alkalosis (or another way of looking at it is an acute respiratory alkalosis that is becoming chronic). The patient's PaO_2 should be at least 380 mm Hg (50 kPa).

Question 13

Chronic respiratory alkalosis. By using the graph, the results lie within this band. By using the arithmetic model, we would expect the patient's actual HCO_3^- to be 15·0 mmol/l. As we can see, the results nearly match this. The slight variance from the predicted results may represent the margin of error for this system or a slight coexisting metabolic acidosis.

Question 14

Acute respiratory alkalosis plus hypoxia. By using the graph, the results lie within this band. By using the arithmetic model, we would expect the patient's actual HCO_3^- to be 21·0 mmol/l. As we can see, the results match this almost exactly. The patient's PaO_2 should be at least 228 mm Hg (30 kPa).

Question 15

Acute repiratory alkalosis. By using the graph, the result lie within this band. By using the arithmetic model, we would expect the patient's actual HCO_3^- to be 20·0 mmol/l. As we can see, the results match this almost exactly.

Question 16

Acute respiratory alkalosis with some compensation, plus hypoxia. By using the graph the results lie off the edge of this band. By using the arithmetic model, we would expect the patient's actual HCO_3^- to be 18·42 mmol/l if it was acute and 10·6 mmol/l if it was chronic. As we can see, the results fall between the two, suggesting that the patient is moving from acute to chronic respiratory alkalosis, with compensation still only partial. The patient's PaO_2 should be at least 380 mm Hg (50 kPa).

Question 17

Mixed metabolic and respiratory acidosis plus hypoxia. By using the graph, the results lie beyond the limits covered by the graph. By using the arithmetic model, for an acute respiratory acidosis we would expect the patient's actual HCO_3^- to be 31·5 mmol/l. As we can see, the result is much lower, indicating a coexisting metabolic acidosis, presumably secondary to the hypoxia. The patient's PaO_2 should be at least 532 mm Hg (70 kPa).

Question 18

Mixed metabolic and respiratory acidosis plus hypoxia. By using the graph, the results lie between the two bands. By using the arithmetic method (for a metabolic acidosis) we would expect the patient's $PaCO_2$ to be 32·6–34·3 mm Hg (4·3–4·5 kPa). As we can see, the actual result is much higher than this, indicating a coexistent respiratory acidosis. The patient's PaO_2 should be at least 380 mm Hg (50 kPa).

Question 19

Mixed metabolic and respiratory acidosis plus hypoxia. By using the graph, the results lie between the two bands. By using the arithmetic method (for acute respiratory acidosis) we would expect the patient's HCO_3 to be 27·71 mmol/l. As we can see, the actual result is lower than this, indicating a coexistent metabolic acidosis. The patient's PaO_2 should be at least 532 mm Hg (70 kPa).

Question 20

Mixed metabolic and respiratory alkalosis plus hypoxia. By using the graph, the results lie between the two bands. By using the arithmetic method (for metabolic alkalosis) we would expect the patient's $PaCO_2$ to be 42·4 mm Hg (5·6 kPa). As we can see, the actual result is lower, indicating a coexistent respiratory alkalosis, presumably as a result of hypoxia increasing the respiratory rate. The patient's PaO_2 is below the expected value for a person breathing room air. The metabolic alkalosis is secondary to hypokalaemia.

Question 21

Metabolic acidosis and respiratory alkalosis, plus hypoxia. By using the graph, the results lie at the junction between metabolic acidosis and chronic respiratory alkalosis. By using the arithmetic method (for metabolic acidosis) we would expect this patient's $PaCO_2$ to be 29·7–32·0 mm Hg (3·9–4·2 kPa). As we can see, the actual result is lower than this, indicating a coexistent primary respiratory alkalosis (presumably secondary to hypoxia). The two primaries have cancelled each other out, resulting in a normal pH. The patient's PaO_2 should be at least 228 mm Hg (30 kPa).

Question 22

Metabolic acidosis and respiratory alkalosis. By using the graph, the results lie between these two bands. By using the arithmetic method (for metabolic acidosis), we would expect this patient's $PaCO_2$ to be 29·9–32·0 mm Hg (3·9–4·2 kPa). As we can see, the actual result is lower, indicating a coexistent primary (iatrogenic) respiratory alkalosis. The two primaries have cancelled each other out, resulting in a normal pH.

Question 23

Metabolic acidosis and respiratory alkalosis plus hypoxia. By using the graph, the results lie between these two bands. By using the arithmetic method (for metabolic acidosis), we would expect this patient's $PaCO_2$ to be 30·5–32·7 mm Hg (4·0–4·3 kPa). As we can see, the actual result is lower, indicating a coexistent primary respiratory alkalosis. The two primaries have cancelled each other out, resulting in a normal pH. The patient's PaO_2 should be at least 228 mm Hg (30 kPa).

Question 24

Respiratory acidosis plus metabolic alkalosis, with hypoxia. By using the graph, the results lie within the band for chronic respiratory acidosis. By using the arithmetic method (for chronic respiratory acidosis), we would expect this patient's actual HCO_3^- to be 33·7 mmol/l. As we can see, the result is higher, indicating a coexistent primary metabolic alkalosis. The two primaries have cancelled each other out, resulting in a normal pH. The patient's PaO_2 is below the normal range.

What has probably happened in this case is that the patient normally suffers from a compensated chronic respiratory acidosis (for example, $PaCO_2$ 70 mm Hg (9·2 kPa)). This produces a compensatory HCO_3^- of 36·5 mmol/l. With the acute infective exacerbation of her disease, however, she becomes hypoxic and increases her respiratory rate, thereby lowering her PaO_2. This produces a posthypercapnoeic metabolic alkalosis.

Question 25

Respiratory acidosis plus metabolic alkalosis with hypoxia. By using the graph, the results lie at the edge of the band for chronic respiratory acidosis. By using the arithmetic method (for chronic respiratory acidosis), we would expect this patient's HCO_3^- to be 30·4 mmol/l. As we can see, the result is higher, indicating a coexistent primary metabolic alkalosis. The two primaries have cancelled each other out, resulting in a normal pH. The patient's PaO_2 is below the normal range.

This is similar to question 24—that is, the patient normally suffers from a compensated chronic respiratory acidosis (for example, $PaCO_2$ 70 mm Hg (9·2 kPa). This produces a compensatory HCO_3^- of 36·5/mmol/l. With the acute infective exacerbation of his disease, however, he becomes hypoxic and increases his respiratory rate thereby lowering his $PaCO_2$. This produces a posthypercapnoeic metabolic alkalosis.

The other possibility is that the patient has a metabolic alkalosis that is compensated for by increasing the $PaCO_2$ (expected value 45·8 mm Hg (6·0 kPa)) but that the infection has produced a primary respiratory acidosis, which raises the PaO_2 further. This is unlikely as there is no reason why the patient should have a primary metabolic alkalosis, also the hypoxic drive would override any attempt to hypoventilate to retain CO_2.

Question 26

Mixed metabolic and respiratory acidosis progressing with treatment to metabolic acidosis/primary iatrogenic respiratory alkalosis. If we look at each sample separately:

Sample 1—By using the graph, the results lie between acute respiratory acidosis and metabolic acidosis. There is no need to use the arithmetic method as the standard HCO_3^- is low and the $PaCO_2$ is high, indicating a mixed metabolic and respiratory acidosis. The patient is also hypoxic (expected PaO_2 532 mm Hg (70 kPa).

Sample 2—By using the graph, the results lie in the middle of the chronic respiratory alkalosis band. In light of the clinical information, we know that this is not the case. If we use the arithmetic method (for metabolic acidosis) we would expect the patient's $PaCO_2$ to be 31·2–33·2 mm Hg (4·1–4·3 kPa). As we can see, the actual result is much lower, indicating a primary (iatrogenic) respiratory alkalosis. The two primaries have cancelled each other out, resulting in a normal pH.

Another way of looking at this is that the compensation for the metabolic acidosis (produced by mechanical hyperventilation) has corrected the pH.

Index